Vagina Revolution

A Candid and Informative Conversation About Vaginas

by

LAURA LEWIN

WITH BARBARA GREEN, P.T., M.S.

Copyright © 2013 by Laura Hankin Lewin

No part of this book may be used or reproduced in any manner without written permission from the author except in brief quotations embodied in articles or reviews.

While writing this book, we checked the scientific information and the latest research. One thing we learned from the research and from many health care professionals is that some information evolves and changes over time. Also not every medical professional agrees on every issue. We tried our best to indicate when that was the case. At this time the information in this book is as up-to-date and as accurate as possible. If anything changes we will be sure to note this on our website www.vaginarevolution.com.

Every reasonable effort has been made to trace copyright holders of material quoted in this book, but if any have inadvertently been overlooked, the author would be glad to hear from them.

Laura Hankin Lewin
[lauralewin@aol.com]

ISBN: 147929912X

ISBN 13: 9781479299126

Library of Congress Control Number: 2012917193
CreateSpace Independent Publishing Platform
North Charleston, South Carolina

Paige —
I feel so lucky to work with you! I hope you enjoy my book!

To Mommy, Daddy, Marc, Max, Kate, and Charlie.

— Laur

Paige -

I feel so lucky I work with you! I hope you enjoy my book!

- Mimi

*I have loved and I have been loved and
all the rest is background music.*

— Estelle Ramey

Introduction

The *Vagina Revolution* has started, and I could not be more thrilled. What began when Eve Ensler wrote and produced *The Vagina Monologues* sixteen years ago has slowly but surely propelled the word *vagina* into mainstream conversation and vocabulary. It has taken years to do this, but just look at what has happened in the past few months—the word *vagina* has been mentioned on numerous mainstream television shows and in movies, thousands of women went to the Michigan state capitol to protest a decision to ban a state legislator from the house floor just because she used the word vagina, and the *Los Angeles Times* printed an article titled "'Vagina,' Once Unmentionable, Has Become a Fashionable Term." Famed feminist author Naomi Wolf even came out with a book recently called *Vagina: A New Biography*.

I am delighted that the *Vagina Revolution* has started in earnest because our vaginas are so important and central to our lives, and yet have been treated badly—we are embarrassed and ashamed of them at worst and ignore them at best. I am excited that vaginas are starting to get their moment in the sun because I have personally been fascinated with vaginas since I was a child, and my awe has only grown over the years. I did not share this particular interest of mine with my friends and family until a few years ago, when I told them that I was starting to research and write a book called *Vagina Revolution*. I was too embarrassed, too ashamed to talk about it. But I had been thinking and wondering for years why so many women felt so embarrassed about their vaginas. I was astonished that so many of us knew so little about our own vaginas. When I was thirty-one years old and trying to get pregnant for the first time, I read a book on fertility because I had been told by many doctors that I would have a hard time getting pregnant because of my diagnosis of polycystic ovarian syndrome. My biggest takeaway from the book was that I could not believe I had come *so far* and yet knew *so little* about my vagina and what came out of it—like cervical fluid, the stuff of fertility. I wanted to share what I had learned with everyone. This made me want to write a book about vaginas to try to demystify and destigmatize them. I figured that if I was unaware of this extremely relevant and important information, perhaps many other women were as well.

My children's favorite movie of all time is *Shrek*. My favorite line from the movie is when Shrek tells Donkey that he (an ogre) is like an onion—he has lots of layers. He uses this analogy to convey that he is complex, and you can't judge him based on his outside appearance. I think this is true about most people, especially women. *We are so very complex.* We have lots of layers. And in order to fully understand us, you need to really take time to get to know us and all our layers.

Vaginas have many layers as well—and I am not just talking about all that wrinkly skin! There is the vulva, which includes the actual vaginal opening as well as the clitoris, labia minora, and labia majora (what we often call the inner and outer lips), as well as the mons pubis. What we collectively think of as our "vagina" is really our vulva, but we have come to call it vagina in our culture, and that is why I do so in this book as well. Another "layer" of our vaginas is interwoven with our minds, which affect so much of what we think about our vaginas. Our minds are influenced by messages we had growing up: What do we think about our vaginas? Are we proud of them or are we embarrassed by them? Or do we ignore them altogether? Vaginas are also intertwined with our spirit and soul. How we feel about issues such as childbirth, gender identity, sexual orientation, and even what is going on with our sisters worldwide affects us on a deeper, more soulful level.

Vaginas are complex and multilayered, but we seldom look beyond the surface because of shame, confusion, and lack of information. Consequently, many women feel a sense of fear and apprehension about their vaginas. Many women have never even looked at their own vaginas. Some women don't even know what *real* vaginas look like. If anything, they only have an image of a picture from a textbook or from porn, and those images surely do not show the wide range of the colors of real vaginas, the beautiful asymmetry of most vaginas. The vaginas in porn are usually one uniform pink color with neat labia, looking nothing like most women's vaginas. It is amazing that women are inundated all the time with pictures of other women's hair, eyes, teeth, breasts, abs, thighs, hips, arms, and so on, but we don't know what vaginas look like. This leads many women to worry about their vaginas looking "normal" and concluding that they do not. Thousands of women even have surgery on their labia so they can look more like those in porn. In fact, labiaplasty is the fastest-growing plastic surgery in many large cities. Even women who are extremely comfortable and at ease with their vaginas and their sexuality often don't know some of the basics—like the names for the different parts of the anatomy, and the huge part they play in their lives.

Introduction

I wrote *Vagina Revolution* not only to demystify and destigmatize vaginas, but also to "normalize" them. It is time for *vagina* to become a household word and not just be whispered in the corner of a room. It is time for women to see pictures of what *real vaginas* look like—vaginas from women of different ages, shapes, sizes, colors, and more. Why does it matter? First, embarrassment and shame over our vaginas just plain feels bad. Any time we hold a negative feeling inside and bury it, it only looms larger, stronger, and more negative. By letting vaginas come out of the closet, we are releasing any negative energy we may have about them, and in turn we will feel better about our vaginas, our bodies, and our sexuality. Also, if we feel less shame and embarrassment, we will be able to talk to our friends about what is going on with our own vaginas and will be better able to talk to our doctors about what is really bothering us. A recent survey conducted by Harris Interactive for the Vagisil Women's Health Center[SM] revealed that although nearly two-thirds of women ages eighteen and older report that they go to a gynecologist, almost one in four of those women (23 percent) admitted that they have not been completely honest about their feminine health habits with their doctors. This survey also confirms the anecdotal statements that many women feel embarrassed discussing their anatomy. The survey revealed that less than half (43 percent) of women indicate that they are completely comfortable discussing their genitals and using the word vagina.[1] When women's fear or embarrassment causes them to lie to their doctors, or to lie by omission—by not discussing something important—it can lead to suffering and undetected medical problems. Additionally, not speaking up about vaginal pain or discomfort leaves us having painful intercourse, when in fact sex should be pleasurable. And being sexual has multiple health benefits—it is right up there with exercising and eating well.

Eliminating the stigma associated with vaginas can help millions of our sisters worldwide, in our own country and across the globe. Vaginas play a huge part in domestic violence, female genital mutilation (two million girls worldwide go through this each year), forced prostitution, and rape. It is estimated that globally, one out of three women will be beaten, coerced into sex, have some kind of trauma to their vaginas, or otherwise be abused in their lifetimes, with rates reaching 70 percent in some countries.[2] The United States and other Western countries are not immune to this mistreatment of women. In the United States,

---

[1] Armen Hareyah, "New Survey Reveals Women's Attitudes About Femine Health," *EMaxHealth*, April 5, 2006, accessed July 2012, http://www.emaxhealth.com/4/5373.html. The poll was conducted by Harris Interactive Poll for the Vagisil Women's Health Center[SM].

[2] Claudi Garcia-Moreno, Henrica A.F.M. Jansen, Mary Ellsberg, Lori Heise, and Charlotte Watts, *WHO Multi-Country Study on Women's Health and Domestic Violence against Women* (Geneva, Switzerland: World Health Organization, 2005).

nearly one in five women surveyed said they had been raped or had experienced an attempted rape at some point, and one in four reported having been beaten by an intimate partner.[3]

I have always been concerned with these issues but having a daughter has opened my eyes to them even more. The other compelling factor that impelled me to write this book was watching my daughter, Kate, as she grew from six to seven to eight to ten years old, and she had so many questions. Some questions were scientific ("Yeah, but mommy, where is the *hole* where babies come out?!") and some were philosophical ("It doesn't make any *sense* that we have to whisper the word of a body part when half the world has that body part..."). Her questions made me ache to change the way that we treat vaginas—the word and the body part. Being around her has opened my eyes even more to women's attitudes about their vaginas and sexuality, and how much this affects women and girls. I am forty-five years old as I write this, and my vagina has gone through a lot since I was a child, including three vaginal births. Society, and the world, has changed since I was a child. We are far more comfortable talking about issues of women's health and sexuality. Information is at our fingertips—we can search the Internet, turn on the television, or even read relevant articles in the *New York Times*. The Vagina Revolution has indeed begun. But the collective energy of guilt and shame about women's sexuality and women's vaginas is still ever present. It is in the air and the water, and we have absorbed it through our pores. It whispers from the back of our minds.

Thus, the revolution. Enough is enough. It is time that women take full control of our cultural attitudes about vaginas and rip to shreds the remaining vestiges of guilt and shame. It is time we fully embrace what is ours—our beautiful bodies and all of our different parts—especially our vaginas. But before this can be fully realized, we need to understand our vaginas from all perspectives—the body (and all of the different parts of our vaginas), the mind (our biggest sex organ), and the spirit and soul of the vagina. We need to get to the point where we do not feel embarrassment or shame.

Vagina Revolution stands on the shoulders of many of my heroes—Eve Ensler, who gave us the *Vagina Monologues*; the Boston Women's Health Collaborative researchers who wrote the classic book *Our Bodies, Ourselves*; sexuality educators like Betty Dodson; organizations that have been educating women for

---

3 Roni Caryn Rabin, "Nearly 1 in 5 Women in US Survey Say They Have Been Sexually Assaulted, *New York Times*, December 14, 2011, accessed July 2012, http://www.nytimes.com/2011/12/15/health/nearly-1-in-5-women-in-us-survey-report-sexual-assault.html. This study began in 2010 and was conducted by the National Center for Injury Prevention and the Centers for Disease Control and Prevention.

Introduction

decades; and so many others who have worked long and hard to bring women's health to the forefront. But our job is still not done. It is my hope that *Vagina Revolution* will help bring us to the tipping point of women's health, safety, and empowerment worldwide.

Vagina Revolution was written to be accessible and fun to read. Reading the book is sort of like eavesdropping on a conversation between two close friends. One of the voices is mine (LL throughout the book) and one is CG, a character who is a *composite expert*. She is mostly based on Barbara Green, a friend of mine whose name is on the cover of this book and who is a physical therapist specializing in work on pelvic floors. But CG also relays a great deal of the information I learned from many of the other women and men I interviewed for the book—OB/GYNs, psychologists, a marriage counselor, a retired midwife, a sex therapist, a gastroenterologist, and my husband, who is a family doctor. It is unrealistic for any one professional to know all the medical and other information put forth in this book, but I do imbue CG with knowledge from the other experts. I also include information from many other experts worldwide with information I gleaned from their informative books and websites.

This book does not need to be read in order—feel free to skip ahead or back to the topics that interest you the most. Nor is the book meant to be a definitive authority on all things vagina; rather it is the start of a conversation that will hopefully spark many other conversations.

I hope you enjoy this book and pass it on to others—your friends, your daughters, your mothers, and even the men in your life. *Vagina Revolution* is meant to give all women a better feeling of control and empowerment over our vaginas and our bodies, and I hope what follows will mean more empowerment in our minds, spirits, and souls. It is time our vaginas come out of the closet and are discussed like any other body part. We are all in this together, and it is time to change the world to make it better, safer, and happier for all women.

If you would like to connect with me or others about any of these topics, please visit www.vaginarevolution.com.

Warmly,
Laura Hankin Lewin
February 10, 2013

Acknowledgements

This book has been such a joy for me to write. I am a school counselor by day, and even though I have a public policy, nonprofit, and research background, I could not possibly have gathered this information without the help of many others. I want to thank the experts who contributed to this book—Barbara Green, a physical therapist who specializes in work on pelvic floors; Dr. Aviva Stein, OB/GYN; Dr. Shraddha Mehta, OB/GYN; Dr. Alyse Kelly-Jones, OB/GYN; Dr. Nancy Teaff, reproductive endocrinologist; Lenore Jones-Deutsch, retired counselor and sex therapist; Marsha Kelly, retired midwife; Dr. Ron Cyzner, gastroenterologist; Matthew Alexander, couples counselor; Dr. Rebecca Fleischer, clinical psychologist; and Dr. Marc Lewin, my husband, my friend, and my love, who is also a family doctor and who fact-checked and helped with everything medical in this book.

I could not have written this book without the help of countless others: my children, Max, Kate, and Charlie, who knew when to let me write and when to ask me to play (OK, they didn't always know this, but they helped me to keep a really great balance and perspective), and my wonderful, supportive friends who only once or twice asked me: "You're writing a book on WHAT?" or "Um, so, what made you want to write a book on vaginas?" in only the way that close friends can ask each other without letting on their complete amazement and disbelief.

A big thank you goes to my friends for reading and commenting on the many drafts or parts of the book: Amy Choffin, Nancy Rones, Cheryl Alley, Lisa Bornstein, Elizabeth Trostler Laban, Rebecca Fleischer, Suzanne Silverman, Barbara Birge, Lauren Abeles, Mara Purcell, Julie Levine, Lenore Jones-Deutsch, Stacey Marshall, Shari Howie, Lori Lucente, Katya Lezin, Clara Irwin, Susan Gundersheim, Marcus Waterbury, Katie Mathis, my wonderful OB/GYN Dr. Sarah Morris, as well as my girls' weekend friends Beth, Debbie, and Becky.

I also want to thank my parents and my brothers for being so supportive. When I first told my mom the topic of the book her reaction was "You're not using your maiden name are you?" She has come a long way since that initial reaction, and now she calls me or e-mails me daily with ideas, suggestions, and offers of help. My older brother, Marc, and my younger brother, Brian, were so helpful and supportive along the way. Marc volunteered his intellectual property law firm to help me trademark the book, and Brian connected me with colleagues in his field to help me with various aspects of the book. I feel so lucky to have had their support and love throughout my life.

I want to thank many others who helped me with different parts of the book: Don Johns, videographer extraordinaire, created a fun and functional book trailer; Jay Cohen, Brian Jackson, and Rob Young did wonderful work on the pictures, diagrams, and graphics; and Betsy Thorpe and Janet Wagner helped tremendously with copyediting. Dr. Marlene Caroselli generously offered to edit some tough parts of the book. Janet Wagner helped with many other details of the book, and I would have drowned in all of the footnotes had it not been for her help. Natalie Ross helped me to keep my message authentic. Sandra Hill at *See The Reaction* designed a wonderful book cover and a perfect website, and Lena Lumelsky at Woland Technology executed it beautifully.

I also want to thank Dr. Robin M. James, associate professor of philosophy and women and gender studies at UNC Charlotte for being my "book whisperer" during the earlier stages of the book.

Barbara Green was a dream to work with. She was extremely knowledgeable, professional, and fun. I absolutely enjoyed collaborating with her on this book.

Lastly, I am grateful to all of my dear friends, family, and colleagues who supported me along the way. I feel so lucky to have you all in my life. You are loving, intelligent, and supportive, and I appreciate each and every one of you. I want to especially thank my loving parents, my sweet children, and my husband who is such a perfect fit for me.

CONTENTS

Part I — VAGINA — THE BODY

1. The Vagina (Hole One) 1
2. The Urethra (Hole Two) 5
3. The Anus (Hole Three) 15
4. The Cervix (Hole Four) and the Rest of the Anatomy 23
5. Hormones 37
6. Vaginal Discharge and Cervical Fluid 43
7. The Clitoris 55
8. The Look of a Vagina 61
9. Smell 69
10. Feel (When Things Just Don't Feel Right) 75
11. Your Vagina Over Time 93

Part II — VAGINA — THE MIND

12. Sexuality and Physical Intimacy 125
13. Masturbation 137
14. Fantasy and Your Biggest Sex Organ — Your Brain! 149
15. Orgasm 167
16. Sex 183

Part III — VAGINA — THE SPIRIT AND SOUL

17. Childbirth and Motherhood 203
18. Sexual Orientation 217
19. Gender Identity 227
20. What Is Going On with Our Sisters Worldwide 237
21. Comfort for the Soul: Taking Care of Your
    Vagina *and* Yourself 259
22. The Word on the Word and the Final Word 267

Foreword

LL (Laura Lewin): I *cannot* remember for the life of me how we got into this conversation, but all of a sudden my daughter, Kate, was yelling "WHAT? You're not allowed to say the word *VAGINA* in an ad on TV? That doesn't make any sense. Everyone comes out of one, so why shouldn't they be allowed to say the WORD?"

Kate has always been obsessed with words. And she is such a curious little thing. I remember when she was five, she asked me how babies were born. I tried to be vague—you know, give her as much information as a five-year-old could digest. I told her that babies grow in your belly, and when they are ready to come out, they are born. That was NOT good enough for her. She kept on pressing and pressing, and finally she said, with a dramatic, exasperated voice, "Yeah, but Mommy, where is the HOLE?" At that point I told her: babies come out through a mommy's vagina.

CG (Our composite expert): You guys are so liberal in your house. My parents never would have told me that when I was that age. I used to think that babies came out of belly buttons when I was a kid. And my parents never bothered to correct me. I think most people wouldn't tell their kids as much as you tell your kids.

LL: My instinct is to tell them the information about what they are curious about. I try to tell them age-appropriate information. If they ask me a question, I might try to get around it if I think they are not old enough to hear all of the details, but if they press, I feel the need to tell them the truth. But I'm always thinking that every child is an experiment. You answer their questions, and you raise them the best you can. The only problem is, you only do the experiment once with each child, and you don't know if it worked until they grow up. And often you don't see how *well* it worked until they are parenting kids of their own.

CG: Well, you have a while to go before that happens. My kids grew up right before my eyes, and they are out of the house; I turn around and ask myself where all the time went. So tell me, what was the big question you wanted to ask me?

LL: Well, I know you do a lot of work with vaginas, that's your area of specialty, and I have been thinking a lot about how little I really knew about my own vagina and my own reproductive system until I was thirty-one and wanted to have a child. This also ties into what Kate was so astonished about. She has asked me many times and in many different ways: if half the population has a vagina, then why is there still so much stigma around and confusion about vaginas?

In the particular case I described earlier, she was referring to a conversation I was having with a friend about a Kotex commercial that was ready to air on TV. The ad had the word *vagina* in it, and three big networks turned down the commercial. Even when Kotex wanted to change the word vagina to *down there*, two of the network television stations still said no to the ad[4]. I was shocked. So was Kate.

So why are so many people still so uncomfortable using the word for that body part on TV? After all, that is what it is—a body part. Why are more than half of women in the United States uncomfortable discussing their genitals and using the word *vagina*.[5] I think that as a society and as a culture we are being so repressed—unless we get more comfortable with the name, and of course the actual body part, we are going to stay in the dark, and our children will grow up repeating the same pattern. Most people avoid the topic. Many women have feelings of shame, discomfort, and embarrassment when thinking about their vaginas. So I was wondering, would you be interested in working on a book to educate other girls and women about what we should know about our vaginas?

CG: You know I love that stuff and would love to talk about this and educate anyone and everyone…but there are already great books out there like *Our Bodies, Ourselves*…

LL: Yes, but I want to make this book short, conversational, and really easy to understand. And I want to have pictures, lots of pictures of real vaginas. As women, we don't even have a good idea about what real vaginas look like. Many of us don't even look at our own vaginas, and if we do, we have no other frame of reference. If we have seen any porn or magazines with pictures, they

---

4 Andrew Adam Newman, "Rebelling Against the Commonly Evasive Feminine Care Ad," *New York Times*, March 15, 2010, accessed February 2012, http://www.nytimes.com/2010/03/16/business/media/16adco.html.

5 Armen Hareyah, "New Survey Reveals Women's Attitudes About Femine Health," *EMaxHealth*, April 5, 2006, accessed July 2012, http://www.emaxhealth.com/4/5373.html. The poll was conducted by Harris Interactive Poll for the Vagisil Women's Health Center[SM].

have certainly always been Photoshopped or airbrushed to look like the *one* kind of standard vagina—the kind that is pink and often prepubescent and has very little hair and perfectly formed labia. The kind of vagina that is presented in porn.

CG: That is a good point. In all of the work I do with vaginas, I don't think I have ever seen the kind of vagina that appears in porn movies or magazines. So often men (and women) get an idea of what women's vaginas *should* look like from porn, and then they pass this on to their partners, sometimes even saying or inferring that their partner's vagina is abnormal when in fact the image of the vagina in porn is more the exception than the rule.

LL: Yet that is what many women compare themselves to. And that is what some men think vaginas should look like. Also, so many women are very self-conscious about their vaginas that there are billions of dollars of products being sold each year to fix what is not even broken. I walked into CVS pharmacy the other day and saw tons of products for women so they could deodorize and douche and get rid of the smell that is actually the natural and healthy smell of a vagina.

The more that women are comfortable with their own vaginas, and the more we can eliminate the nervous energy we have around vaginas, the more free we will feel, and the less self-conscious we will be, not to mention the more educated.

CG: OK, so what should we do? List the most important things every woman and girl should know about their vaginas?

LL: Yes. And include pictures of real, live vaginas from women of all ages, colors, nationalities, body types, weights, and so on.

CG: Because my area of specialty is to work on pelvic floors, I do a lot of work inside women's vaginas to help them with one issue or another such as birth trauma or painful intercourse. So many women are so often self-conscious, scared, and embarrassed. I tell them, "They all look different and they all look normal!" But then they start with the questions: Is my vagina discolored? Is it weird that it is asymmetrical…I mean one lip is so much bigger than the other one? What is the sticky stuff that comes out of my vagina?

LL: This is what I am talking about. Could you help me to list the answers to many of these questions that women have?

CG: Absolutely. You know I am always up for talking about vaginas. Let's get started.

CHAPTER 1

The Vagina (Hole One)—The Star of the Show!

LL: So where do we start?

CG: OK, let's jump right in. Now, we have lots of holes in our body, right? We have a mouth, a hole in each ear, two in our noses, and so on. We need all of these holes to live, to experience the world, and to reproduce. So speaking of that, let's talk about the holes in the area of our vulva. Look at this picture of a thirty-five-year-old woman's genetalia.

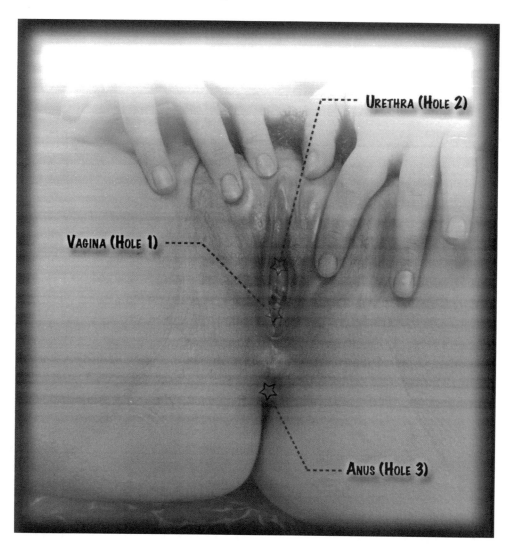

If you look closely you can see three holes. I love how your daughter asked about where the hole is where babies come out because, of course, there has to be a hole if something is coming out, or going in, for that matter. So let's examine the holes. We will go from smallest to largest.

The smallest one is sort of hidden. It is called the urethra (hole two). That is where urine comes out. The medium-sized one is called the anus (hole three), and that is where feces (poop) exits the body. And the largest of the holes (hole one) is called the vagina (the opening into the vaginal canal is the *introitus*), and that is where menstrual blood comes out, as well as babies when they are born. It is also where penises and sperm and tampons and anything else go in. It is the passageway from the uterus and cervix (more on those two later) to the outside world. The vagina is framed by the inner and outer labia. There will be more on those parts of the anatomy in chapter four but for now, you can look at the picture on the next page. Collectively the whole area is called the vulva, or external genetailia.

LL: I thought the whole area was called the vagina.

CG: No, actually the area shown in this first picture is called your *vulva*. Many people use *vagina* to refer to what is really the vulva.

LL: So maybe we should call this book the "Vulva Revolution."

CG: Well, technically it should be, but our culture has come to know the whole shebang as the vagina, including the actual opening, which is part of the vulva.

If you look in a medical dictionary, it will say that the vulva consists of the external genital organs of the female mammal. This includes the *mons pubis* — the *mound* above the vagina that is soft and fleshy and where most of your pubic hair resides. The vulva also includes the clitoris (that is actually hidden in this picture, but it is above the holes and below the mons pubis). The clitoris gets its very own section later in the book.

Here is a close-up picture so you can see the parts even more clearly.

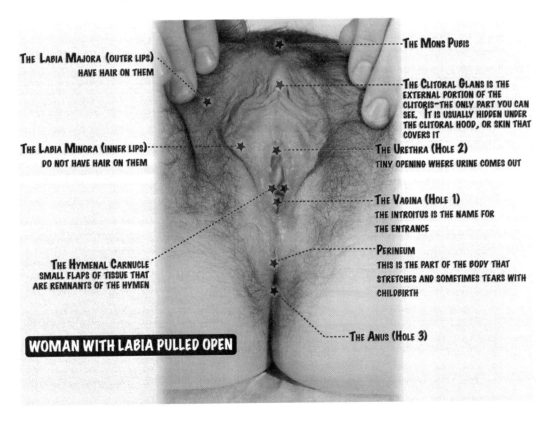

Now look at the part that is labeled vagina (hole one); that is the vaginal opening. Even though we call it the vagina, technically the vagina doesn't start until after the opening.

The vagina is essentially the passageway part of the vulva. It is an elastic, muscular canal that has a soft and flexible lining. Think of the vagina as a hallway from the outside entrance (the vulva and the labia) to the uterus (where babies grow). The hallway is usually collapsed (sort of like a glove is collapsed until you put your fingers in it, and then it expands to fit your fingers). The muscle in the vagina passageway expands to let things in (for example, tampons) or out (for example, babies).

LL: So the vagina is just a narrow, empty passageway made of muscle?

CG: Yes—it expands and contracts depending on what is in there. It also secretes lubrication, and the whole area is a place of great sensation for most women.

LL: So when I get a yeast infection, that is in hole number one, right?

CG: Exactly. That is important to point out because yeast infections are so common. Seventy-five percent of all women get at least one yeast infection in their lives. (See the chart in chapter two on what infections you get in what holes, what causes the infections, and how you can prevent them.)

Join the Revolution: *Know All of Thy Body Parts!*

Just *knowing* all the anatomy of your vagina, the other anatomy in the region, and where all the parts are located, puts you way ahead of the game. Make sure to pass this information on to friends, your daughters, sisters—even your mother. Give them the quiz on the vaginarevolution.com website. The more we know about our vaginas, the more comfortable we become, and the more empowered we are to address any issues we have with our vaginas. The more comfortable we are with the body part and the word, the more positive energy we have surrounding our body.

CHAPTER 2

The Urethra (Hole Two)

CG: Hole number two is the urethra. This is a tube that connects the bladder to the outside world so our bodies can get rid of urine. Look at the picture labeled Urethra (hole two). The urethra in women is fairly short because it only has to go from the bladder to right above the vaginal opening and right below the clitoris. Men have a urethra, too, but it is longer because it has to go down the length of the penis. Men have just one hole that you can see, and both urine and semen travel through this one passageway.

Vagina Revolution

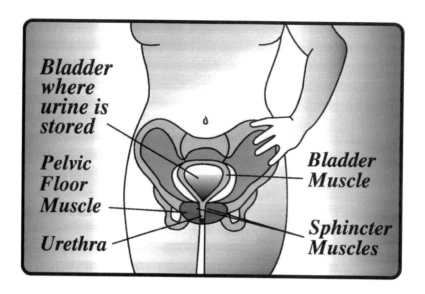

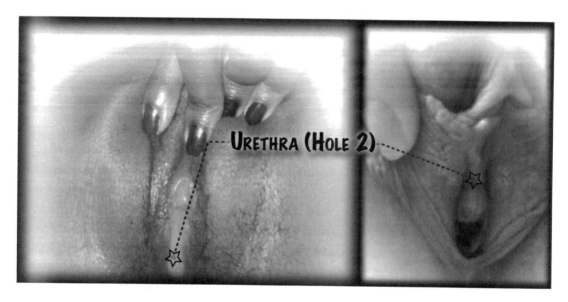

LL: Hole number two sounds much less complex than hole number one.

CG: True, but it still serves a very important function because when you gotta go, you gotta go. But also because the urethra is often the entrance point for bacteria that cause those darn UTIs—urinary tract infections.

LL: Ugh—I used to get those all the time, especially when I was younger. This book really isn't about medical conditions per se because there is so much to say about them, and it would make this book way too long. But since UTIs are so prevalent, can you please share some basic information about the most common infections women get?

CG: Sure. I will list the three biggies and some medical information about all three—yeast infections (found in the vagina—hole one), bacterial vaginosis (also found in hole one), and UTIs (found in the urethra—hole two).

One important thing that all women should know about their urethra is that they should monitor their urine—check the color, the smell, and the volume. The color of urine may change throughout the day, from a dark yellow first thing in the morning to pale yellow or even colorless if a woman is drinking a lot of liquids during the day. When a woman's urine is dark, and it is not the first thing in the morning, that can indicate that she is not drinking enough water.

The color of urine can also be affected by what you eat—for example, if you eat a lot of beets, your urine can look pinkish. The bottom line is that a woman should get to know what her urine looks like and smells like for health reasons. If there is a change, it might indicate that something is going on, and it is time to visit a doctor to investigate.

LL: What about smell? I notice that my urine smells different in the morning than at other times of the day.

CG: That is also normal, and it goes along with the darker color urine in the morning. There is more concentrated urobilin in your urine in the morning. It is important to know the normal smell of your urine because if you happen to notice that your urine smells "funny" or very different, and/or you have pain or a burning sensation when you urinate, go see your doctor right away. Chances are you have a UTI or something else, and you may need to be on an antibiotic. But your doctor can tell you for sure, and it is not worth waiting and risking a worse infection.

Some women never or rarely get UTIs, while others can't seem to keep them away. On average UTIs are very common. About a third of all women in the United States are diagnosed with a UTI by the time they are twenty-four years old. In fact, UTIs are the most common infectious disease in women, accounting for 8.1 million visits to health care providers in the United States each year.[6]

---

[6] S.M. Schappert and E.A. Rechtsteiner, "Ambulatory Medical Care Utilization Estimates for 2006," National Health Statistics Reports, No. 8 (Hyattsville, MD: National Center for Health Statistics, 2008).

This is huge. Hundreds of millions of women worldwide get UTIs each year.[7] For women, the lifetime risk of having a UTI is greater than 50 percent.[8]

LL: Why do so many women get UTIs, and how can we prevent them?

CG: One reason why women get UTIs so easily is that a woman's urethra is fairly short, allowing bacteria quick access from the anus or vagina to the bladder. Many women get UTIs because foreign bacteria often goes up into the urethra during sex.

LL: Hole two?

CG: Yes, and if bacteria from someone's hands or penis travel up the urethra, that can cause a problem.

LL: Are there other symptoms of a UTI besides pain or a burning sensation when urinating?

CG: Some women also get a fever or pain in the lower abdomen, back, or sides. Many women have a strong urge to urinate, and yet very little urine comes out and sometimes it could be tinged with blood. On average women should urinate anywhere from seven to nine times a day, or every two to four hours. If a woman notices an increase in her normal frequency, coupled with other symptoms mentioned above, then she may suspect a UTI. If you experience any of these symptoms, it is important to see a doctor to get tested for a UTI. The danger in waiting is that the infection could progress into something worse like a kidney infection, which is much more serious.

LL: Is there any way to prevent UTIs?

CG: I always recommend urinating after sexual intercourse because if any bacteria are trying to climb up your urethra, you flush them out before they even have a chance. I also recommend drinking plenty of water, approximately eight glasses a day (this recommendation depends on where you live, how active you are, and other factors). Always wipe from front to back so bacteria from your anus don't get near your urethra. And avoid feminine products that could be irritating like douches, powders, and sprays.

LL: I have another question. I also hear so much about yeast infections, and I used to get those all the time, too. How are they different from UTIs?

---

7 Tomas L. Griebling, "Urinary Tract Infection in Women," in *Urologic Diseases in America*, M.S. Litwin and C.S. Saigal, eds. (Washington, DC: GPO, 2007), 594, accessed September 2012, http://kidney.niddk.nih.gov/statistics/uda/Urinary_Tract_Infection_in_Women-Chapter18.pdf.

8 Ibid.

CG: Well, now we are back to hole one because you don't get yeast infections in hole two.

In hole number one, your vagina, you have lots of natural fungi that normally live in the vagina in healthy amounts. You also have a normal pH level, a level of acidity. But sometimes something causes these fungi to grow, and this overgrowth is what we know as a yeast infection. Also sometimes the normal pH level changes and this causes the normal level of good bacteria and bad bacteria to become unbalanced and this leads to another condition called bacterial vaginosis (BV).

BV could be caused by something you do to upset the pH balance in your vagina. For example, you may think that douching is harmless, but it actually washes out a lot of the good bacteria from your vagina and changes the pH level in your vagina. These changes can also make your vagina a good environment for yeast to grow and overgrow, and this can also cause a yeast infection.

Yeast infections can also be caused by something going on with your health, including taking antibiotics. Usually women do not get yeast infections as a result of sex, but it could be from a weakened immune system.

Yeast infections are more likely the result of increased stress in your life, and as you know this always has a big impact on your immune system as well.

And yeast can be passed back and forth between sexual partners, but this is rare.

Symptoms of yeast infections include itching and burning in your vagina or it could be a funny smell or a discharge that can look a bit like cottage cheese.

LL: Gross!

CG: No, it's not so gross, but it is something that women definitely need to address. About seventy-five percent of all women get a yeast infection at least once in their lives.[9] Symptoms may be different for women as they get older. They may have more global symptoms like feeling flushed and sweaty, which could mean many things. Also older women may be more prone to yeast infections if they are using hormone replacement therapy.

LL: Can you please sum up the difference between UTIs, BV and yeast infections?

---

9 HHS Office of Women's Health, "Vaginal Yeast Infections: Frequently Asked Questions, Sept. 23, 2008, accessed June 2012, http://www.womenshealth.gov/publications/our-publications/fact-sheet/vaginal-yeast-infections.pdf.

CG: Sure—check out this chart. But also please remember: Do not self-diagnose. I know that there are some over-the-counter medications, but women are often wrong about their self-diagnoses, and they can overlook a sexually transmitted infection or something else. **So when experiencing any of these symptoms, please see a doctor or healthcare professional!**

	YEAST INFECTIONS[10]	**BACTERIAL VAGINOSIS (BV)**[11]	**URINARY TRACT INFECTIONS (UTI's)**[12]
LOCATION:	Hole #1 – Vagina	Hole #1 – Vagina	Hole #2 – Urethra
SYMPTOMS:	Burning, redness, and swelling of the vagina and vulva; Painful urination and or sex; Discharge looks white and clumpy, similar to cottage cheese; Symptoms may be mild or severe	Most women with BV report no signs or symptoms at all but some describe discharge, pain, itching, burning, or a fishy odor that is more noticeable during menstruation or after sex	Burning during urination; Frequent urge to urinate even if there is only a small amount to pass; Pain in lower back or side, may be accompanied by fever and chills; Cloudy, dark, or foul smelling urine
OCCURRENCE:	75% of women get at least one	29% of women ages 14-49 have had BV; BV is the most common vaginal infection for women of childbearing age—16% of pregnant women are estimated to have BV	11% of women have a UTI at any given time

---

10 http://www.womenshealth.gov/publications/our-publications/fact-sheet/vaginal-yeast-infections.pdf.
11 http://www.cdc.gov/STD/bv/STDFact-Bacterial-Vaginosis.htm
12 http://kidney.niddk.nih.gov/statistics/uda/Urinary_Tract_Infection_in_Women-Chapter18.pdf.

The Urethra (Hole Two)

CAUSES:	Yeast is a type of fungus that lives naturally in vaginas—a yeast infection occurs when there is an overgrowth of yeast. Causes include: stress, lack of sleep, too much sugar, hormonal changes, certain medications such as antibiotics, pregnancy, or diabetes	When the normal balance of bacteria in the vagina is disrupted and replaced by an overgrowth of certain bacteria; Douching; Many sexual partners (women who have no sexual partners may also get BV)	Bacteria travels up urethra. A culture must be taken to officially determine if bacteria are present in the urine
PREVENTION:	Wear cotton underwear; Change out of wet bathing suits; Sleep without underwear; Avoid tight clothes; Change pads and tampons frequently; Avoid douches; Avoid scented hygiene products	Do not douche; Use condoms and limit the number of sexual partners	Urinate after intercourse; Drink lots of fluids; Wipe from the front to the back; Wear cotton underwear and loose-fitting clothing; Drink cranberry juice (there are conflicting studies about this)
TREATMENT:	Over the Counter antifungal medications or prescribed medication	Antibiotics prescribed by doctor; Male partners do not need to be treated but female partners do	Antibiotics prescribed by doctor; Studies show that two-thirds of women who self-diagnose are wrong!

LEVEL OF CONTAGION:	Not a Sexually Transmitted Infection but yeast can be transferred to partner, though it is rare	BV may spread between female partners	Not contagious
MYTH:	Not caused from having sex, rather a weak immune system or other causes listed above		Not caused by bad hygiene

- ❖ Some of these symptoms are similar to symptoms of some sexually transmitted infections…if you experience any of these symptoms see your doctor.

Join the Revolution: *Pull Out Those Vagina Mirrors!*

Do not shy away from *looking* at your vagina. What kind of message are you sending to yourself if you can't even look at this important body part? And what kind of message are you sending your brain about how much you like your vagina? Are you embarrassed by it? The more you study it and know what it looks like, the more comfortable you will become with it.

Know exactly what your vagina looks like. And love it. Send it messages like "You are beautiful," or "I love you and appreciate you." And THANK your vagina for doing so much for you in your life. If not for your vagina, you might not experience as much pleasure in life.

The Urethra (Hole Two)

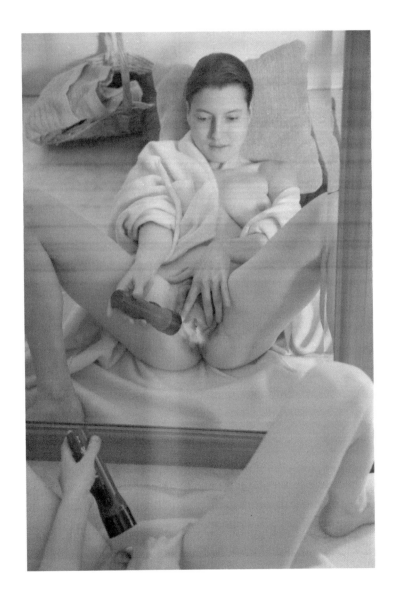

CHAPTER 3

The Anus (Hole Three)

LL: I debated long and hard about including hole three in this book, or at least about giving it a lot of prominence and its very own chapter.

CG: I think it is important. I have had patients who have mixed up all the holes and still have confusion. And a lot of younger people often ask about the difference between the holes. So while technically it is not part of the vulva, I think it is a very prominent and important place in the region.

[CG is a composite expert but sometimes she morphs into one of the specialists/experts. She is now morphing into a gastroenterologist] Now let's look at this third picture. This woman is forty-three years old. Notice that the anus has a brown color that gets a bit lighter as it goes out for a few centimeters, until it blends in with the buttocks.

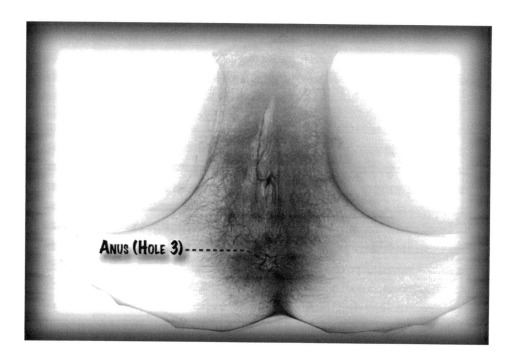

LL: The cheeks.

CG: I prefer the word *buttocks*, but you can use whatever term you feel most comfortable with.

LL: Speaking of hole three, I have a question I have wondered about for a while. I remember this *Oprah* episode a few years ago where Dr. Oz was talking about poop and what it should look like at its healthiest. It made a big impression on me. I felt like for days I heard people talking about what poop was supposed to look like and what it was not supposed to look like. For example, Dr. Oz said that your poop should come out in a soft but formed "log" and not balls. I remember him explaining what he meant by balls. He used the term "plop, plop" — the sound the poop makes when it hits the water in the toilet.

CG: Yes — there can be a big difference in what feces looks like. I didn't see that episode but perhaps he was talking about the Bristol Stool Scale[13]?

---

[13] Bristol Stool Scale or Bristol Stool Chart is a medical aid designed to classify the form of human feces into seven categories. Sometimes referred to in the UK as the Meyers Scale, it was developed by K.W. Heaton and S.J. Lewis at the University of Bristol and was first published in the *Scandinavian Journal of Gastroenterology* in 1997.

LL: What is that? And why does it really matter how your poop comes out?

CG: Your feces say a lot about how you have been eating and your bowel habits. If you have been eating enough fiber and drinking enough water, and if you have been getting a fair amount of exercise, then your feces should come out like a log. You should not have to force it out and you should not have to push hard. You should be able to feel when your body is ready to move its bowels, and just let your body do the work without much added pushing.

And as for the Bristol Stool Scale, this is a medical aid to help doctors and others classify human feces into seven different types. Here are the seven types:

1. Type 1: Separate hard lumps, like nuts (may be hard to pass)
2. Type 2: Sausage-shaped but lumpy
3. Type 3: Like a sausage but with cracks on the surface
4. Type 4: Like a sausage or snake, smooth and soft
5. Type 5: Soft blobs with clear-cut edges
6. Type 6: Fluffy pieces with ragged edges, a mushy stool
7. Type 7: Watery, no solid pieces, entirely liquid

Types one and two indicate constipation, while types three and four are the more ideal stools because they are easy to defecate while not containing any excess liquid. By the way, if you would like to see descriptive pictures you can easily find them online. The Bristol Stool Chart even has its own Facebook page!

LL: Can you please tell me how often you are supposed to poop? I have heard different people say different things.

CG: "Normal" is considered anywhere from three times a day to three times a week. It is important for women to be aware of their own pattern of when they move their bowels and pay close attention to it. **If your pattern changes, it is important to discuss this with your doctor.**

LL: Do you mean it could indicate that something is wrong?

CG: It could be something simple like your pattern changes when you are under stress or traveling.

LL: Yeah, I rarely poop the first few days when I travel.

CG: However it could also indicate an underlying issue. Same thing applies to when you wipe and find blood on the toilet paper.

LL: That used to happen to me a lot when I used to get constipated.

CG: It is common to find blood on the toilet paper when you wipe, in fact thirteen percent of people occasionally find blood on the toilet paper when they wipe.[14]

LL: I can't believe they do studies about that!

CG: If you ever find blood on your toilet paper, this is something you really should get checked out by the doctor. Most often the cause is something simple. Hemorrhoids bother about eighty-nine percent of all Americans at one point in their lives. Hemorrhoids are a swollen blood vessel on the rectum. They look like bumps the size of peas or sometimes bigger. Bleeding can also be caused by a fissure, which is a tiny cut at the edge of your anus.

LL: What is the difference between the anus and rectum?

CG: The anus is the hole—the actual opening where the feces come out. The rectum is the area right inside the hole. It is the final, straight portion of the intestines, and it terminates in the anus. The rectum is where your feces are stored. When the rectum is full, it signals your body that feces are ready to come out, but if you don't act on that urge, then the feces are often returned to the colon, where more water is absorbed. Sometimes, not going for a long time can cause constipation. That's why it is very important to act on the urge to defecate whenever you feel it.

Here is a diagram of all of the parts:

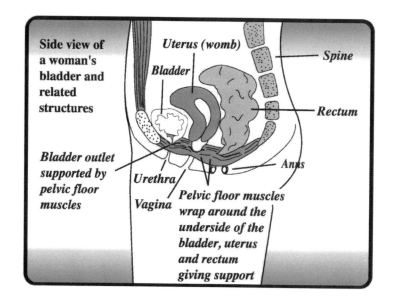

---

14 N.J. Talley and M. Jones, "Self-Reported Rectal Bleeding in a United States Community: Prevalence, Risk Factors, and Health Care Seeking," *American Journal of Gastroenterology* 93 (1998) : 2179.

If you follow the tube up a bit farther past the rectum, you will find the sigmoid colon and then the rest of the colon. The food that you eat goes into your mouth and travels through your gastrointestinal tract—the twenty- to thirty-foot tube extending from your mouth to your anus. As the food moves through, your body absorbs important nutrients from it. The rest gets processed in your colon and comes out as feces (or waste product) through your rectum, and then out through your anus. There is a muscle called the anal sphincter that allows the anus to open and close. When the sphincter opens, it allows the anus to let out the feces and then closes up again. Just a quick note on the word sphincter: there are other sphincter muscles in your body as well, including the urethral sphincter which allows your urethra to open and close to let out urine.

LL: Is there something wrong with me if I feel like I need to poop, and then I have to make a run for the bathroom?

CG: You should be able to delay going to the bathroom once you have the urge to defecate. For example if you are in your car, you should be able to drive home or to a rest stop, calmly walk to the toilet, and go to the bathroom. You should be able to wait about thirty minutes. At the same time, if you do feel the urge, and you are near a bathroom, then you should not ignore your urge. The sensation of the stool in the rectum is your body's way of telling you it needs to defecate, and we should always listen to our bodies as best we can.

LL: I have one more big question. Can you please tell my readers and me some of the most important things about poop, and maybe include what your patients are curious about?

CG: Sure! One, it should be brown in color. It can change colors, but if it changes too much (for example if it is green, that means there is too much bile in your feces), and if that change occurs for more than a day or so, then you should tell your doctor. If it is gray or tarry black or if there is blood in your feces, those things can all indicate something is not right, and again, you should tell your doctor. But usually, if there is a change and a couple days later it goes back to normal, it might just mean you had a virus or something else transient that has resolved by itself.

Two, it takes approximately one to three days for your food to enter your body and then come out the other end. Your body takes the important nutrients out of the food, and then sends the rest to the wastebasket. Some people digest food more quickly than others—sometimes as quickly as eight to fourteen hours. If you want to see how quickly you digest food, you can always do the *corn test*. Eat some corn and monitor your feces for the next few days. Since some whole kernels of corn pass through your system, you can see the kernels in your feces and thus see how long your system is taking to digest food.

Third, feces are supposed to smell! There are trillions of bacteria in your gut that break down the food and turn it into what we see coming out on the other end. It is good for it to smell, it just means the bacteria are doing their job well.

LL: OK, let's all thank the bacteria in our gut.

CG: As we discussed earlier, everyone has a different pooping pattern. Some people poop three times a day, and some people move their bowels three times a week. As long as this is your personal norm, then there is nothing wrong with it. But if someone is not defecating at least three times a week, then I think she should consult with a doctor. And if she is constipated, then she should increase her fiber intake — most people should be eating between twenty and thirty-five grams of fiber a day. The average American only eats half the fiber she needs. If you are eating about five servings of fruits or vegetables a day, as well as six servings of grain products per day (at least three of which are whole grains), then you are probably eating enough fiber.

Eating fiber is extremely good for your health in many ways, including your digestive health. Additionally, eating fiber softens dense poops and solidifies wet poops — it fixes everything.

And you need to drink a lot of water — *not soda or caffeine* — hydration is very important. And of course exercise. When you exercise, you increase the motility (movement) of stool through your colon, and you generally tend to move your bowels more frequently.

LL: OK, is there anything else?

CG: Gas!

LL: Gas? You mean my eight-year-old's favorite topic of conversation?

CG: Yes — kids have the right idea. Don't hold it in. Let it all out. It feels bad when you hold it in. Of course, not if you are on a first date or in an important meeting with your boss. Then you really should hold it in, and you should *be able to* hold it in. If you cannot hold in your gas, then you may have gas incontinence, and you should go to see a doctor. Many older people have gas incontinence because muscles weaken with age. But there are things you can do at any age to strengthen your pelvic floor muscles and lessen gas incontinence.

When it comes to gas in general (with these exceptions in mind) then I say let it out. Depending on what you eat or if you are constipated or not, your gas

The Anus (Hole Three)

does not always smell. If it does, it might mean you are eating too much food that does not agree with you and perhaps you should examine your diet. You should be passing gas between ten and twenty times a day. If you hold it in, it just makes you feel gassy and bloated. So let it out!

LL: My kids are going to love hearing that one. Not that they have ever had a problem holding back.

CG: Before I leave, I have one more thing to say to your readers. As a gastroenterologist, I would be remiss if I did not add this to a book about women's health issues. Everyone—women and men—should get a diagnostic colonoscopy at age fifty, or earlier if they have a family history of colon cancer. So many Americans and others around the world have gotten colon cancer with very few symptoms. This is a very serious and very deadly kind of cancer. It strikes one hundred and thirty thousand Americans each year, and fifty-five thousand of those Americans, a quarter of them under the age of fifty, die from it.

LL: I remember when Katie Couric's husband died from colon cancer. He was only forty-two years old. I hadn't realized until then what a serious kind of cancer it was. He didn't have symptoms—or rather, he didn't realize that he had symptoms. I read that he had been very tired, but he was also traveling a lot, and he was a busy professional—who isn't tired?

CG: So true. I thought it was amazing, too, when Katie Couric went on national television to have a colonoscopy to show how easy it was and also to make the point that the more people who get colonoscopies the better the chance of preventing colon cancer. If everyone went in for a colonoscopy it would prevent between sixty and ninety percent of all deaths from colon cancer. That is between thirty thousand and forty-five thousand lives saved in the United States alone.

CHAPTER 4

The Cervix (Hole Four) and the Rest of the Anatomy

LL: I didn't really realize that there was another hole. Where is it?

CG: This one is a little bit tricky. If you travel all the way up hole one, the vagina, inside you will find the cervix. The cervix is the opening to the womb (uterus). The cervix plays a very important role during pregnancy and labor. During pregnancy, the cervix remains closed and blocked with a mucus plug. This keeps anything harmful out of the uterus so the baby can safely grow inside.

If a woman has never had a baby, then the cervical opening is very small. It could even be the size of the head of a pin, though it needs to be big enough for menstrual blood to come out or sperm to go in.

After a woman has delivered a baby vaginally, the opening of the cervix is permanently changed. It now looks more like a slit, though the internal junction between the cervix and the uterus is closed. If you look at the next picture and examine the cervix, the fleshy mound at the center of the picture, you can actually see the slit that I am talking about, labeled as the external cervical os.

The cervix is remarkable in so many ways. First, it protects babies by not allowing anything through to the uterus. Think of all of the weight that sits on it, and the pressure that it must endure, and it still remains closed. Even if the outer hole starts to open up toward the end of pregnancy, the inner part of the cervix stays closed.

And speaking of the end of pregnancy, when a woman's hormones shift to prepare for delivery, the hormones cause the cervix to thin out, to shorten, and to open slightly. The cervix gets softer and turns a bluish color. During labor, the cervix goes from being a very small hole to ten centimeters (about four inches) dilated so that the baby can come out of the uterus and through the cervix, down the vagina and out into the world.

Check out these two images and imagine the cervix in the first picture opening up to let out a baby. You can see the baby's head coming through the cervix in the diagram on the next page.

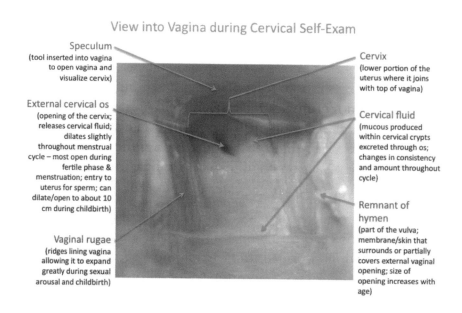

The Cervix (Hole Four) and the Rest of the Anatomy

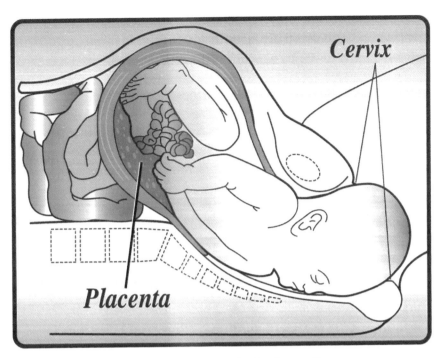

Cervix (Hole 4): the teeny tiny hole that allows sperm to go in and babies to come out of the uterus...when the cervix dilates to 10 centimeters a woman can usually start pushing the baby out of her uterus and through the cervix, and out through the vagina.

LL: Wow—what a miracle. That very small pinprick of a hole opens up to let out a whole baby.

CG: If you've had a baby, and the doctor checked your cervix to see if you were dilated, or if the hole was open wide enough for the baby to start coming out, then it was hole four that she was checking. When she says, "Oh, you're only two centimeters dilated. Come back in a week," then that little hole on top of the small hill in the first picture[15] is not a pinhole any more. It's really an opening the size of the diameter of a quarter. But a baby still cannot fit through that. At ten centimeters dilated, that little pinhole is now the size of an orange, and it's time to start pushing out that baby. And all of that happens behind the scenes, before the baby even makes her way through the vaginal canal.

I don't want to leave out an important part of a woman's anatomy. At the other end of the uterus are the two fallopian tubes—one going to each ovary. Eggs

---

15 Thank you to Beautiful Cervix Project for giving us permission to reprint this image. Accessed September, 2012 http://www.beautifulcervix.com/your-cycle/

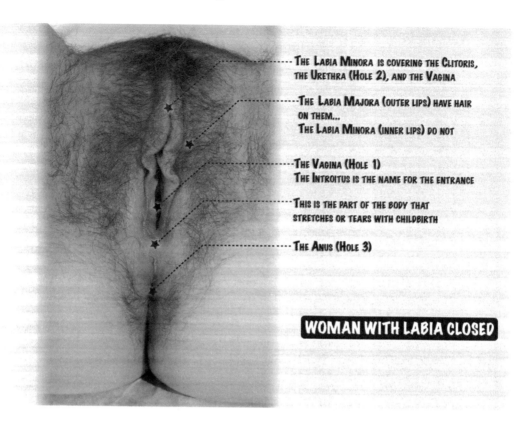

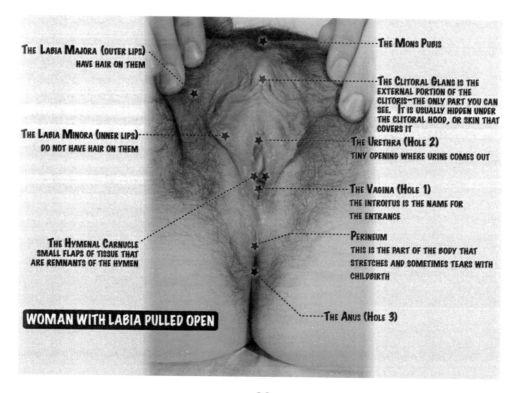

originate in the ovaries and then travel down the fallopian tube. The sperm swim up through the cervix and the uterus to meet the egg in the fallopian tube. We could talk for hours about the miracle of pregnancy, but let's stick to your original question about the vagina for now. We will just touch on the surrounding anatomy.

I marvel at all four holes, as I do at the rest of the anatomy in our vaginas.

LL: I, too, am in awe. And there are still other parts of the genetalia we have not even examined yet. Can you please label the rest of the parts? I want to make sure I get them all right…like outer lips and inner lips — how can you tell them apart?

CG: Sure — check out the two pictures below, which are clearly labeled.

The Labia

Do you see the outer lips? Those are called the labia majora. The inner lips are called the labia minora. One way to tell them apart is that the outer lips have hair, and the inner lips do not.

One important fact about the labia (especially the inner labia) is that they are often different sizes — women may have labia that are often asymmetrical, meaning that one side or lip can be larger than the other side.

Look at the montage of picture, below. You can see the variety of labia and how some of them are uneven. This is completely normal. Come to think of it — I would say that most of the labia I see are asymmetrical, sort of like a woman's breasts are often different sizes.

Sometimes this can bother women. Some of my clients are embarrassed by it. But it is *so, so common.* I see it *all* the time.

If having large labia bothers a woman for a medical reason, for example if her labia brush against her underwear and chafe during exercise, or if her labia cause her to have painful intercourse, then there is a surgery to repair this. The surgery, called labiaplasty, can help fix the irritation or pain in some cases. But I only recommend this surgery in extreme cases.

I also caution against this surgery and tell my patients only to get it if they know all the risks. Short-term complications of labiaplasty include bleeding, bruising, swelling, infection, and scarring. Long-term complications could include a loss of sensation (especially if a woman is "trimming" or surgically removing some of her labia); spotting; difficulty urinating; change in pigmentation, usually along the edges of the labia; and separation of the incision site.

Vagina Revolution

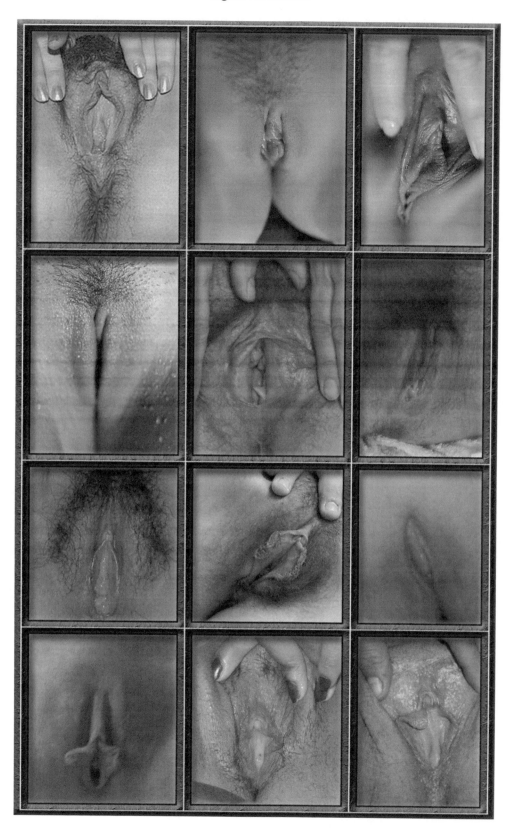

Just as with everything else, a woman has to weigh the risks and rewards of any surgery. If her labia are a constant source of irritation, then it might be worth it to have surgery.

LL: What about labiaplasty for aesthetic purposes — I have heard that this is the fastest-growing plastic surgery in some cities.

CG: I don't like to think about that because I am biased. I have seen so many vaginas, and they are all so unique. To me unique is a good thing — like petals of a flower or snowflakes or people's faces. So I don't like when women say they are going to get surgery to "fix" their labia, when they are really not broken, just different. Every woman's labia are different, unique, and therefore beautiful.

LL: Maybe all women should just agree that labia can be different shapes and sizes, and we should appreciate our unique differences. Just like our ears are different shapes and sizes (mine are two completely different sizes), and most women have two different-sized breasts — there is no reason to be embarrassed by the way our labia look.

CG: Amen, sister.

Join the Revolution! *Love Thy Labia!*

OK, so breasts are aesthetically pleasing, right? Men can't stop staring, and countless artists have drawn them as objects of beauty or sexuality. So what about labia? Labia have been in the closet for so long (although they have been celebrated by artists like Georgia O'Keefe and Nick Karras — see http://www.nickkarras.com/ or http://www.ilovemypetals.com). Labia can be perfectly imperfect. More often than not they are asymmetrical. More often than not they have shaded coloring. Let's embrace them, no matter what their color, shape, or size. Don't try to change them to look pink and prepubescent. Labiaplasty (also known as vaginal rejuvenation) has led to some lawsuits because no one factors in the pain and discomfort that often comes along with unnecessary surgery on such a sensitive body part.

Join the revolution and embrace the fact that labia are beautiful as they are.

The Mons Pubis

Look at these two pictures, above. What do you notice?

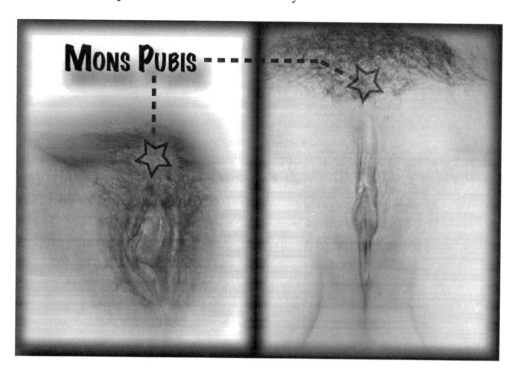

LL: I notice that in both vaginas you can't see the actual opening of hole one or hole two. Also, the labia are different sizes. And I notice hair. Although it looks like in the picture on the right the woman has shaved her hair so that it is only on the top and not the sides of her vagina.

CG: Exactly! So that is the next place I want you to look. Do you see the *mound* where the hair is in the second picture? That is called the *mons pubis,* and it is sometimes shortened to mons. It is the cushiony, often triangular mound that sits above a woman's vulva and is covered with pubic hair. This cushiony area protects the woman's vagina in many ways—for example, it protects the delicate organ beneath during sex.

LL: What do you mean protects it?

CG: Imagine a woman having sex with a man who weighs much more than she does, and he is on top. When he moves inside of her or when he lies on top of her, his weight is fairly well distributed so he doesn't crush her. When their two genitals meet, there is a lot of pressure and disproportionately more weight that would fall directly on the vagina. Thankfully, we have a built-in cushion—our mons!

If you look directly under the mons, you will see a small, raised mound surrounded by the top of the labia minora and the clitoral hood. That is the clitoris. It is usually hidden under the clitoral hood. I am only going to quickly point out the glans of the clitoris and then move on because the clitoris gets its very own chapter later on.

The G-Spot

LL: I have always read in books and women's magazines that women have a G-Spot. But there seems to be so much controversy and confusion over this. Why is that?

CG: It's no wonder that you are confused. The G-Spot, which was named after German gynecologist Ernst Grafenberg who did research in the 1940s, has been studied as far back as the 1600s, but there are still experts who argue for and against its existence, its location, and its function. And there are conflicting studies that come out about it all the time. Honestly if you put two medical experts in a room to talk about G-spots they will probably emerge with three different opinions.

LL: How would you define it—assuming you think it is real?

CG: I do think it is real. There is way too much evidence and way too many women who say it is real. But I don't think it is real for all women.

I know many women who swear that it is real and that it is fabulous. And I know other women who swear that they don't have a G-Spot. Or they spend years looking for it, and they are frustrated by their efforts. I know others who say they only discovered their G-Spot after having their first or second or third vaginal birth.

The G-Spot is a ridged area on the upper front wall of the vagina, near the urethra and under the pubic bone. It is defined as a bean-shaped area of the vagina. When stimulated, it can lead to sexual arousal, powerful orgasms, and female ejaculation in some women.

LL: If a woman doesn't know where it is and wants to try to find it, or see if she has one, then what should she do?

CG: Most women report that they feel their G-Spot approximately two to three inches inside the vagina on the anterior, or front wall, the wall closest to your belly button. Some women claim if this spot is stimulated, they can have a more intense orgasm than with clitoral stimulation. However it is a difficult area to reach because if a woman is having sex in the missionary position (man on top), his penis does not stimulate the G-Spot area. It requires stimulation from different angles, from fingers, or from vibrators or sex toys.

For some women the G-spot is very sensitive and for others less so. It is similar to nipples in this way—some women like the feeling of having their nipples stimulated and others do not. I absolutely encourage exploration in this area. There are some videos on YouTube and many books to help women figure out if they have a G-Spot and if so, where to find it.

The Hymen

LL: I know you are not done yet, but I want to ask you to talk about the hymen. It's one part of a woman's body that has been the cause of lots of pain, some physical but mostly emotional, in so many cultures throughout history.

CG: Sure. If you look at the drawing below, you will notice that there is a thin membrane or a sliver of smooth, crescent-shaped tissue that *partly* covers the vaginal opening. Can you see that?

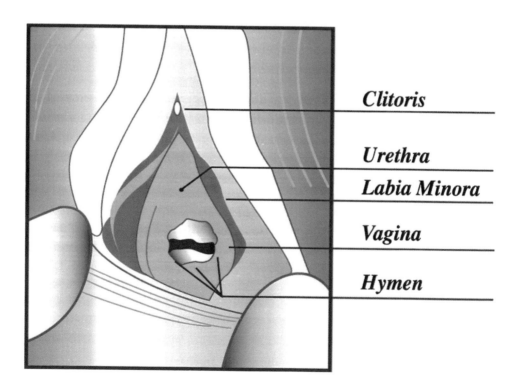

LL: Yes.

CG: Hymens come in different shapes. Sometimes when a woman's hymen has been broken you can no longer notice the shape, but you may notice that it looks like another crease or wrinkle at the bottom part of the vaginal opening. Some women are predisposed to have more stretchy hymens, and some women are genetically predisposed to have more taut hymens. And some women have no noticeable hymen at all.

In the normal course of life, the hymenal opening can also be enlarged by tampon or menstrual cup use (a cup you can insert in your vagina to collect the menstrual blood), pelvic examinations with a speculum, regular physical activity, or sexual intercourse. Once a girl reaches puberty, the hymen becomes elastic and estrogenized, and it is not always possible to determine whether a woman is a virgin by examining her hymen. And sometimes it is possible to determine that a woman is a virgin if the hymen is still prominent.

Knowing all this, here is the big hype about the hymen. In many cultures all over the world, an intact hymen is highly valued at marriage mainly to "prove" virginity. In some cultures, there is someone assigned to examine the potential bride to determine if she is a virgin. In other cultures, the community waits around until the marriage is consummated to see if there is any blood on the sheet. The blood supposedly shows that the intact hymen is now broken and has bled from the bride's first intercourse.

LL: Whoa! This is starting to raise the hair on the back of my neck here. To have a woman's private parts examined when there is not a male equivalent is a terrible double standard. I know that this is practiced in many places in the world, including some places in the United States, but the double standard really bothers me. And like you mentioned, *sometimes when you do look at a woman, you can't tell if she is a virgin anyway.*

CG: Exactly. Although the practice is common, it is not really possible to confirm that a girl or woman is a virgin by examining her hymen.

Also in one survey, only forty-three percent of women reported bleeding the first time they had intercourse, indicating that the hymens of a majority of women had already opened through everyday activities.[16] And sometimes bleeding occurs from the stretching of some veins or blood vessels in the vagina

---

16 Astrid Heger, S. Jean Emans, and David Muram, "Physical Examination of the Child and Adolescent," in *Evaluation of the Sexually Abused Child: A Medical Textbook and Photographic Atlas*, 2d ed. (New York: OUP, 2000), 61–65.

when it is stretched out for the first time, but this bleeding is not necessarily from the hymen.

LL: In many cultures, if a woman is not a virgin, then no one will want to marry her. And in some cultures, the fear of being caught having had premarital sex, or the fear of not having a noticeable hymen, even if the woman truly is a virgin, leads women to undergo a surgery called hymenoplasty to replace their hymen so that their communities will still see them as virgins. I find this incredibly offensive and unfair.

CG: We don't want to be disrespectful of the standard for any culture or group. Also sexual activity is and should be a very personal decision. I have seen many women who have waited to have sex until marriage and they can have very healthy sex lives. I have also seen many women who have had multiple sexual partners before marriage and they can also have very healthy sex lives.

There have been books and articles and reviews written about this concept. Being a virgin is a topic that is also debated in our own culture. If you want to learn more about this I recommend reading *The Purity Myth: How America's Obsession with Virginity Is Hurting Young Women* by Jessica Valenti.[17] You can also find an interesting, quick analysis of the history of hymens at http://www.answers.com/topic/hymen-10.

---

17 Jessica Valenti, The Purity Myth: How America's Obsession with Virginity Is Hurting Young Women, (Berkeley, CA: Seal Press, 2010).

> ### Join the Revolution: *End the Hype Over the Hymen!*
>
> The teeny-tiny sliver of skin at the entrance to the vagina, the hymen, has been used throughout time and across cultures to judge if a woman was a virgin or not. Women are born with hymens of different shapes and sizes, and it is not possible to tell if a woman has had sex or not by simply looking at her hymen. Many women stretch out their hymens by using tampons or through horseback riding or other activities. Judging a woman by looking at her hymen is unfair for many reasons. First, it is a double standard: there is no body part to check on a man to see if he is a virgin or not (and anyway, it is usually not a requirement for marriage). Second, checking a woman's hymen is not an accurate, sure-fire way to see if she is a virgin, and in many cultures women have suffered because someone falsely claimed they were not virgins. In some cultures, the fear of being judged as someone who has had sex before marriage has led many women to get unnecessary surgeries to create hymens just so they can prove that they are virgins. Many women are pressured to avoid sexual intercourse (penis-in-vagina) before marriage but are simultaneously pressured to engage in other types of sex acts (anal or oral). Is that unfair or what?
>
> Enough is enough! It is time we end the hype over the hymen for once and for all. It is no one's business if a woman is a virgin or has a defined hymen except for that woman—and anyone with whom she *chooses* to share this information.
>
> Millions upon millions of women have been subjected to unwanted people looking at their vaginas and passing judgments on their hymens, and untold thousands have been punished based on this. This is cruel, humiliating, and unfair.

Suggested Resources:

Bachman, Barbara. *Our Bodies, Ourselves for the New Century: A Book by and for Women.* Boston Women's Health Collective, ed. 4th ed. (New York: Touchstone, 2005).

This is a classic and a must-have resource for all women!

Rankin, Lissa. *What's Up Down There? Questions You'd Only Ask Your Gynecologist If She Was Your Best Friend*, (New York: St. Martin's Griffin, 2010).

> Lissa Rankin's book was one of the first books I read after deciding to write *Vagina Revolution*. I was inspired by Lissa's ability to make the topic of vaginas so friendly and easy to read. Lissa also has a wonderful blog—http://www.owningpink.com/blogs/lissa-rankin.

CHAPTER 5

Hormones

CG: I like to describe all the anatomy like the holes and the labia and hymen as the *hardware* of the vagina and the hormones as the *software*. The hormones help the different parts communicate and relate to one another and the rest of the body. The hormones tie the parts together. They're what make the parts work with each other as a whole.

LL: I'm a middle school counselor, so when you say the word *hormones*, I cannot help but think of my students. I deal with hormones every day. I have four hundred and twenty students, so it is not surprising that I get a lot of kids crying in my office. I have been with the same kids for three years now — through the sixth, seventh, and eighth grades. I know these kids really, really well. So I can pretty much tell every month or so when someone bursts out in tears *for no reason* that it is usually because some hormone is wreaking havoc on his or her body without prior warning. I am also pretty sure that hormones are the culprit when a child starts acting out or experiencing test anxiety, social anxiety, or general jitteriness.

But the crying-for-no-reason thing especially shouts out to me, "Major hormonal change happening here!"

Sometimes when this happens, it makes me think that maybe *we are all* just a collection of hormones. And I wonder if maybe we have no free will — we were preprogrammed to do what our bodies tell us, and we are the way we are because of our hormones. But that is a discussion for another day.

CG: In some ways this is true. Our hormones are very much affected by our genetics, and they do rule so much of our lives. Hormones affect so much in our bodies — not just sexual arousal and the reproductive cycle. Hormones also stimulate or inhibit growth; activate or inhibit the immune system; regulate metabolism and cause hunger cravings; prepare the body for mating, fighting, and fleeing, as well as for new phases of life such as puberty, parenting, and menopause; and much, much more.

LL: When it comes to the vagina, is there any way you can explain all of these crazy hormones and what they do?

CG: Sure. I will give a brief overview of hormones in women. Since this is just an overview, I will only briefly mention the reproductive system — that is a whole book on its own — and concentrate on how hormones affect our vaginas and the surrounding region.

Brief Overview of Hormones

Hormones are chemical substances made naturally in your body, and secreted from endocrine glands throughout the body. Hormones are your body's chemical messengers, moving mostly through the bloodstream, regulating the way other organs, tissues, and structures function. There are approximately thirty-seven different kinds of hormones that can be found in women, and they are all responsible for doing different things. They work slowly, over time, and affect many different processes, including[18]:

---

18 For more information on hormones, see http://www.nlm.nih.gov/medlineplus/hormones.html.

- Growth and development
- Metabolism – how your body gets energy from the foods you eat
- Sexual function
- Reproduction
- Mood

The major endocrine glands are the pituitary, pineal, thymus, thyroid, adrenal glands, and pancreas. In addition, men produce hormones in their testes, and women produce them in their ovaries.

Although there are thirty-seven different hormones, some hormones have a greater effect on women, including estrogen, progesterone, and testosterone. These hormones are made in a woman's ovaries, the small almond-shaped sex glands in the pelvis that also produce a woman's eggs.

The ovaries are active during fetal development, but they become relatively inactive throughout infancy and childhood. When a girl starts getting ready for puberty, the ovaries become very active again, and they start to produce adult sexual development and urges, as well as the mood swings we all associate with puberty and PMS.

Adolescent hormone production comes in fits and starts. Anyone who has or who has had an adolescent can confirm this! The hormones are irregular until the body figures out the precise amounts. That is probably what is happening to your students who come to see you after bursting into tears. After puberty, most women settle into a more or less regular pattern of ovulation.

The ovaries make estrogen and progesterone, as well as various other hormones and the levels of these hormones rise and fall with ovulation. Ovulation is when the egg is released from the ovary. This day is typically fourteen days counted from the first day of menstrual bleeding, though this is based on an average twenty-eight day cycle. Some women have irregular periods and others have longer than—or shorter than—twenty-eight day cycles. Most women ovulate every cycle from puberty until perimenopause or menopause (more on that in chapter 11). Ovulation is interrupted by pregnancy, nursing, and even by stressful events.

<u>Estrogen</u> is considered to be the primary female hormone. During puberty it causes breasts to grow and vaginas to mature. Specifically it builds up the uterine lining and thickens the vaginal wall. It also affects almost every other organ in the body. Estrogen plays an important role in bone building and is thought to have essential protective effects on the cardiovascular system.

Progesterone, which is made only during the second half of the menstrual cycle, prepares the uterine lining for an egg to implant. Progesterone also has important effects on many of the tissues sensitive to estrogen. Progesterone has been associated with decreased sexual desire in women though this is not yet fully understood. Testosterone, also made in the ovaries, plays a role in stimulating sexual desire, generating energy, and developing muscle mass. Testosterone is better known as a male hormone,[19] but women have it naturally too, just in smaller amounts.

The hormone oxytocin is also implicated in female sexual motivation. It is a hormone that is released at orgasm and also during breastfeeding. Oxytocin is associated with both sexual pleasure and forming close human bonds.

The system of hormones in our bodies is very complex, and the balance of hormones in your body is affected by many factors. The pituitary gland, at the base of your brain, and your ovaries are constantly communicating by way of their respective hormones, dictating the changing hormone levels of your monthly cycle and the production of eggs. The pituitary produces follicle-stimulating hormone and other hormones. *Stress, body weight, time of day, time of the month, and any medications you take can all cause temporary changes in your hormone levels.*

Menopause brings major, permanent changes to the hormone levels and hormone balance of your body. The ovaries stop releasing eggs, and they also decrease the levels of hormones they produce. This does not happen all at once. By their late thirties, many women are producing less progesterone, which can lead to heavier, more frequent periods early in the *perimenopause* process. Then the ovaries' estrogen production tapers. It is the fluctuations in estrogen production and, later, the decrease of estrogen that primarily brings on the discomforts and health concerns associated with menopause.

How Hormones Affect Your Vagina
If you only take one piece of information out of this section, it should be this — estrogen keeps the vaginal walls healthy and lubricated.

On the other extreme, at menopause, when there is little estrogen stimulating the vaginal wall, the vaginal walls tend to get dry. As a result some women experience painful intercourse, as well as general pain and discomfort in their vaginas even when not having intercourse (more on that in chapter 10).

---

19 Many people argue that hormones should not be known as "male" or "female" hormones because we all have different levels of all these hormones.

Hormones are also one of the big factors that affect a woman's *sexual response* (it's actually a very complex interaction of biology/hormones, and sociocultural and psychological factors).

When a woman is sexually aroused, her hormones—primarily estrogen—cause an increased blood flow to the clitoris and the vulva. Some women describe this feeling as feeling "engorged" or "full." This blood flow also causes a woman's clitoris to double in size because the erectile tissue fills with blood and becomes, well, erect.

LL: Just like a man's penis.

CG: Right—both men and women have *erectile tissue* in their genitals.

The estrogen also causes vaginal *transudation* or the seeping of moisture through the vaginal walls, which will serve as lubrication. Also, the woman's vagina enlarges inside to better accommodate a penis or fingers or a vibrator.

Stimulation of the woman's clitoris or vulva or other areas also leads to more engorgement and lubrication. There is an increased redness or darkening of the skin in the whole vaginal area. A woman's heart rate and blood pressure also slightly increase, and she may feel hot or flushed.

If sexual stimulation continues, the sexual arousal may peak in an orgasm. After having an orgasm, many women do not want any further stimulation, but some may want to continue. Some women may experience second or third or more orgasms.

Another hormone, oxytocin, is released when a woman has an orgasm, and it is associated with both sexual pleasure and the formation of emotional bonds.

CHAPTER 6

Vaginal Discharge and Cervical Fluid

Vaginal Discharge

CG: Some more "software" that interrelates with your "hardware" is something called vaginal discharge. It includes all the fluids that come out of your vagina.

LL: Do we have to use the word *discharge*? I mean it is such a negative word. It sounds like something that is being rejected.

CG: It is not! I never think of it as a negative word. It's just the word that everyone calls the natural stuff that comes out of your vagina. Women ask me about it all the time.

LL: You mean the stuff that can pool in your vagina at night and in the morning drips down your leg? The stuff that gets in your underwear, and you need to hide it from your partner or die of embarrassment with the old middle school joke ringing through your ears "that's as old as the crust in your underwear"? The stuff that pantiliners are perfect for catching? (Though using pantiliners is not a good idea on a daily basis—more on that later.) The stuff that has prompted every woman at one point or another to go to the doctor to ask if she has a yeast infection?

CG: Ha! I hear that question all the time. Yes, that stuff. This liquid is called vaginal discharge, and it is natural and normal, just like the saliva in your mouth and the tears in your eyes.

LL: Now you tell me. I wasted a very good co-pay over that many years ago.

CG: I cannot tell you how many patients I have seen over the years who come in worried about what is coming out of their vaginas. Most of the time it is just good, normal, healthy discharge. Vaginal discharge is fluid made by glands inside the vagina and cervix. It serves a great, helpful purpose by carrying away dead cells and bacteria. This keeps your vagina clean and protected from infection.

Vaginal discharge is sort of the catch-all name for a bunch of different liquids that flow from your vagina. Your vagina is a mucous membrane. It is similar to the mouth and the nose in this way, and a common analogy for the vagina is that it is like a self-cleaning oven.

From Lissa Rankin's *What's Up Down There? Questions You'd Only Ask Your Gynecologist If She Was Your Best Friend:*[20]

<u>What is vaginal discharge made of? Is it toxic waste or something?</u>

No, it's not toxic waste. In fact, unlike urine and feces, it doesn't contain any waste products. What it does contain is:

- Fluid that seeps through the walls of the vagina
- Cervical mucus
- Uterine and tubal fluid
- Secretions from glands in the vulva

---

20 Lissa Rankin, *What's Up Down There? Questions You'd Only Ask Your Gynecologist If She Was Your Best Friend* (New York: St. Martin's Griffin, 2010), 152-153.

> - Oil and sweat from vulvar glands
> - Old cells from the walls of the vagina
> - Healthy bacteria
>
> Your vaginal discharge consists mostly of salt water, mucus, and cells—things that normally exist in your body. There's really nothing icky about it. Vaginal discharge helps maintain a healthy system.

But sometimes, especially if your vaginal discharge is accompanied by itching, pain, a burning sensation, a change of color, or a funny smell, then it could indicate a yeast infection or bacterial vaginosis or some other kind of infection. When in doubt, always see a doctor.

Cervical Fluid

Cervical fluid is one of the most noticeable kinds of vaginal discharge. Cervical fluid is different from the natural lubrication that forms in your vagina when you are sexually excited. Cervical fluid is the mucus that is secreted from the cervix and produced by the hormone estrogen in the first phase of a woman's menstrual cycle.

Cervical fluid is a key part of fertility and a woman's ability to get pregnant. Cervical fluid actually helps the sperm find its way to an egg. Just like semen, cervical fluid acts as a medium for the sperm and helps transport it to the egg. PLUS the cervical fluid filters the sperm and only allows the morphologically normal sperm to proceed. Furthermore, the cervical fluid nurtures and supports the sperm biochemically AND protects it from the acidity in the vagina—sometimes for up to five days while waiting for a woman to ovulate. Increased cervical fluid may also increase a woman's lubrication. The increase in cervical fluid is triggered by the same hormonal cycle that promotes ovulation, and when both happen at the same time, this may correlate with an increase in a woman's libido. This is one of the reasons why women feel a higher sex drive when they are ovulating—when they are at their most fertile.

LL: Wow, how fascinating.

CG: Cervical fluid changes over the course of the month (or however long your cycle is), and the changes happen when your hormones change. So after your period is over, and the bleeding stops, most women don't have much fluid coming out of their vaginas. The vagina is usually dry-ish. By the way, you can see the fluid when you wipe, if you look at the toilet paper, or if you gently insert a finger into your vagina and feel whether it feels wet or dry. A few days after your period ends, you might notice some sticky cervical mucus. If you put it between your pointer finger and your thumb, and then you open and close your thumb and finger, it will feel a bit sticky—almost like a trace of maple syrup. You might even start noticing this on your underwear.

As you get closer to ovulation, you might notice a change in the cervical fluid. It gets creamy and looks and feels sort of like lotion. Then when you ovulate, the fluid gets very slippery and stretchy and resembles egg whites. If you take the fluid and stretch it between two fingers, over the course of a week you will see that the cervical fluid is the stretchiest during the most fertile time in your cycle.

LL: Here is a great picture of a woman's cervical fluid at the most fertile point in her cycle.

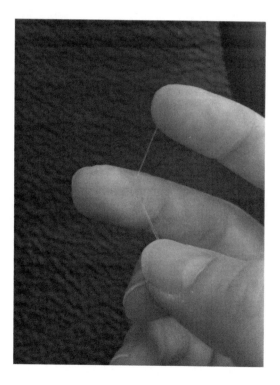

CG: One time I had a patient come to see me who was very embarrassed. She said it was like she had a watery version of that kid's toy called slime that was practically flowing from her vagina and running down her leg. She was not happy about that one bit and was very anxious about it. Do you know what her condition was? *Fertility*! I told her that, and she almost ran me over to get home to her husband because they had been trying to conceive, and they thought she was fertile at a different time of her cycle.

LL: I remember learning about this when I was thirty-one and trying to get pregnant. I can't believe I didn't know about it before that.

Last summer I had a chance to educate someone about cervical fluid. I was going to lunch with a good friend of mine whom I only see once or twice a year. We both work full time. I have three kids, and she has one. Also, she is a very serious, successful professional. At lunch last summer, I asked if she and her husband, Bob, were planning to have another child, and she confided in me that they had been trying for two years but had not been successful. I wanted to ask her if she knew to check her cervical fluid so she could tell when she was fertile. I tend to get embarrassed much less than your average person, but just as I was about to ask her, I started to doubt myself and felt embarrassed.

And then I thought to myself "Well, suppose she doesn't know to examine her cervical fluid to see when she is most fertile…and suppose this piece of information could help? But then, chances are she does know because she is so smart and successful, and she has been having fertility issues for two years." I really didn't want to say anything, but I am so glad I did. It turned out she didn't know about cervical fluid — she was completely in the dark like so many of us — and it did make a difference.

CG: So she's pregnant?

LL: Due this July!

CG: That is a great story. And it shows the power of one woman sharing information with another.

LL: It's what we do best in so many other areas — suggestions for what to make for dinner, food that kids will like, problems with our bosses, debating whether to go back to work or stay home, taking care of our elderly parents, signing kids up for different activities…We share tons of information every day, yet vaginas are taboo, even with close friends. That is part of why it is time for vaginas to come out of the closet. We will be more comfortable sharing information not only about fertility, but also about sexuality and anything else that is going on with our vaginas.

CG: I could not agree more.

Menstrual Blood

LL: Now what about blood—the other liquid that comes out of your vagina? Is there anything new and interesting that we should know about our periods?

CG: There is so much to say about menstruation, but I think most women are pretty familiar with the basics. I will just mention a few things here. For the basics, I definitely recommend reading *Our Bodies, Ourselves.*

As women remember from their health classes in school, each month in preparation for pregnancy, the lining of the uterus, also referred to as the endometrium, thickens to prepare for fertilization and implantation, and is then shed, resulting in a bloody discharge. The sloughed-off lining leaves the uterus, moving through the cervix, and out of the body through the vagina.

So many women complain about their periods because, let's face it, who wants blood flowing out of her vagina for four to six days each month for thirty-plus years of her life? It is messy. Sometimes it comes on when we are unprepared. BUT (and this is a big but), just like everything else in life, we can either find things to complain about or we can find the blessings—the silver linings. When we can think about those things, we change our entire attitudes. We are LUCKY that we menstruate. We should thank our bodies every time we menstruate because it is a sign that our systems are working.

Second, menstrual symptoms and all the moods that accompany our cycles do not have to take us by surprise. When I was growing up, I discovered a "secret" my parents had. My father would track my mother's cycle by writing on a note card that he kept in his top dresser drawer. He would write down the day of the month, starting on the first day of her period, and he would write little notes to himself like mom was going to be "moody and cranky" on days twenty-six and twenty-seven of her cycle, for instance. I bet he stayed away from her or at least trod very lightly on those days.

When I was twelve and got my first period, I started doing this for myself. Not only did I track my moods, but also the feelings associated with those moods. I remember at the beginning of my period I felt a big relief, and I felt really good about everything. Then somewhere in the middle of my cycle—probably when I was ovulating, but I did not know that in those years—I would feel very creative and spend a lot of time on my drawings. After that, during maybe the third week or so after my period, I had a day or two of sadness and one day of *extreme* self-consciousness. Sometimes I also felt unappreciated or unloved. Then, sometime around when I got my period, I felt really, really happy and relieved. And one of my physical symptoms, which I also charted, was that I would always be constipated for a few days, but then poop the day I got my period.

After a few months of charting, I recognized a very cyclic pattern. My cycle has always been forty-two days long, but even though my cycle was longer than most, my moods and other physical symptoms were like clockwork. The great thing about charting was that I didn't feel like I was taken by surprise by intense feelings or emotions because I could always predict what day they were coming. Even though the feelings felt very real, I could look back at my charts from different cycles and see that everything was pretty darn predictable. And then I could tell myself that a certain intense feeling I was having was just part of my cycle—what I now understand to be part of a hormonal cycle.

LL: Let's recreate this chart and put a copy in the appendices (see appendix 1). I'll also put it on the website as a Word document so women can screen grab it and put in their own person-specific changes that they notice—or if they want to turn it into a fertility chart or add some notes about their diet and changes in hunger or anything else, they can do that as well. And there are even Apps for charting out there!

> ### Join the Revolution: *Fully Understand Your Own Cycle*
>
> I mean *fully* understand. Do you know on what day of your cycle you get cranky? On what day you are most creative? On what day you are positive that everyone dislikes you, and you have no friends left in the world? And then what is the day when nothing can spoil your great mood? What day you are bloated and stopped up? There is so much in your life that follows the same cycle as your menstrual cycle (postmenopausal women and men have hormonal cycles, too). This can include not just your mood, but also the amount of cervical fluid coming out of your vagina, and how hungry, tired, or energetic you are. This could include how sensitive your breasts are. How easily aroused you feel—or not. CHART all of this so you can have an excellent handle on your moods, energy, health, and cyclical changes. This can empower you to plan certain events, dates, or meetings on certain days and plan a good mental-health day on another day in your cycle. Or it can just make you feel better, if you are having one of those no-one-loves-me days, to go back and see that this is falling on the same exact day of your cycle as last time. That realization can be *priceless.*

> How do you figure all this out? Spend three to four months charting ALL your changes. Use the chart on the vaginarevolution.com website or at the back of this book, or simply create your own. You will notice that the same changes happen on the same days of your cycle month after month. Menstruation, ovulation, thin or slippery cervical fluid, sticky or tacky cervical fluid, and smell—your vagina might be odorless at one point in your cycle, and smell musty during another point. You may notice that your bowel movements follow this cycle, too. Maybe even the kinds of foods you crave, the mucous in your nose, the amount of energy you have may follow this cycle. Share this information with your partner so he or she can be more supportive (or stay away from you) on your "cranky" day but ask you for help on a project during your "creative" week. Know when you are going to feel lazy so you can ramp up your exercise beforehand. Basically, this helps you to understand yourself and to know that so much of what you feel at any point is actually hormonally controlled.

CG: Most of us think about two basic options for catching the blood that flows from our vaginas—commercial tampons or pads (also called sanitary napkins). Using a product worn outside your body (such as a pad) or inside it (such as a tampon) is a matter of personal preference. But there are inventive new products that women can try that they may prefer.

For example, a company in Britain developed a menstrual cup called the Mooncup, which you can insert into your vagina to catch or collect the blood and then dispose of it in the restroom.[21] The Mooncup is being marketed to women who want to help the environment. The company says that the cotton in most sanitary products contains pesticides and bleaches, and a total of 4.3 billion sanitary products per year end up in landfills in Britain. (Plus they have a great website and a great song titled "Love Your Vagina!")

I also just read about another menstrual cup called Lunette on a blog I like called *Because I Am a Woman*.[22] The blogger, Ally Boguhn, writes that she likes Lunette better because it comes in different colors, is smaller and more pliable,

---

[21] Mooncup, *Love Your Vagina*, accessed June 2012, http://www.loveyourvagina.com/index.php/index/static#.
[22] Because I Am a Woman (blog), accessed January 11, 2013, http://becauseiamawoman.tumblr.com/post/22689105719/lunettereview.

and the website has easier directions. She does mention that one advantage of the Mooncup is that it is larger, so women with heavier flows don't need to take it out and rinse it as frequently. There are also other brands of menstrual cups available, including Diva Cup, Soft Cup, and Instead.

Other women prefer to use washable cloth pads. Some women opt for organic, washable fiber. Both of these options are also cost-effective and good for the environment.

LL: Do you get a lot of questions about the consistency of menstrual blood? I remember being in my early twenties and looking at a blood clot that came out of my vagina and being shocked that it could be so big, and frankly, so scary looking!

CG: Yes, I get that question all of the time. So most periods last between three and five days, but the range is more like two to eight days. And on average only four to eight tablespoons of blood come out, but boy, can that seem like much more when it's soaking through tampons or pads.

Many women have an occasional clot in their menstrual blood. The clots may be bright red or dark in color. Often, these clots are shed on the heaviest days of bleeding. The presence of multiple clots in your flow may make your menstrual blood seem thick or denser than usual.

Your body typically releases anticoagulants to keep menstrual blood from clotting as it's being released, but when your period is heavy and blood is being expelled rapidly, there's not enough time for the anticoagulants to work. That enables blood clots to form.

If you have excessive clotting or clots larger than a quarter, you should see a doctor to rule out any conditions that might be causing an abnormal period such as endometriosis or fibroids.

Sometimes you may notice that your menstrual blood becomes dark brown or almost black as you near the end of your period. This color change is normal. It happens when the blood is older and not being expelled from the body as quickly.

You should not worry if your flow is temporarily heavy, but if you regularly have heavy periods, I would suggest seeing a doctor and making sure your blood count is normal. If you soak one sanitary pad or tampon per hour several times during a twenty-four-hour period, your flow would be characterized as heavy. If this is happening, even if it is something you are used to and you think is normal, see a doctor to make sure your blood loss is not so high that you become anemic.

CG: Birth control pills allow women to control the length of their periods. The bleeding from a pill period is different from bleeding caused by your own hormonal shifts. I, for one, like to menstruate each month, but if women don't want to have their periods as often, there are other birth control options out there that will stop them from menstruating as frequently. They should ask their doctors about these options, which include taking birth control pills back to back without taking a break.

LL: Before we move on to the next chapter, I want to go back to something you mentioned earlier. What is wrong with pantiliners?

CG: I wouldn't say you should never wear a pantiliner. They are awesome if you just had sex and need to get dressed and go do errands…or go to work or on the very light days of your period. They absorb tons of liquid—much more than seems possible given their slim size. But I think it is very important for vaginas to be able to "breathe" more. When you are wearing a pantiliner, it holds moisture right up against your labia and vulva, and the more moisture in your vaginal area, the better the environment for yeast or bacteria to grow. Dr. Elizabeth Stewart's *V Book: A Doctor's Guide to Complete Vulvovaginal Health* explains that pantiliners are not recommended for daily use because they hold moisture close to the skin for too long, and they can be abrasive.

I love that Dr. Stewart says "It is far better to change underpants several times a day if you have a lot of normal discharge. This may be the case during pregnancy, for example, or this may be the normal state for you. Remember that a little wetness or a yellowish stain on your underwear is not a sin. It's normal."[23]

I recently read this great quote by an OB/GYN who goes by Dr. Kate on her website[24], "We have this notion that we need to be bone-dry, all the time (except if we're aroused. Then we can't be too wet). But a little discharge on your vulva is OK—moisture keeps you from sticking or chafing. So don't wear liners to protect your panties—wear panties to protect your clothes (which is actually what underwear is *for*). Just change them during the day if you feel the need."

---

23 Elizabeth Stewart, *V Book: A Doctor's Guide to Complete Vulvovaginal Health*, (New York: Bantam, 2002), 96.
24 Dr. Kate, "Why Pantiliners Are Evil," *Gynotalk*, August 12, 2009, accessed December 2011, http://www.gynotalk.com/2009/08/why-pantiliners-are-evil.html.

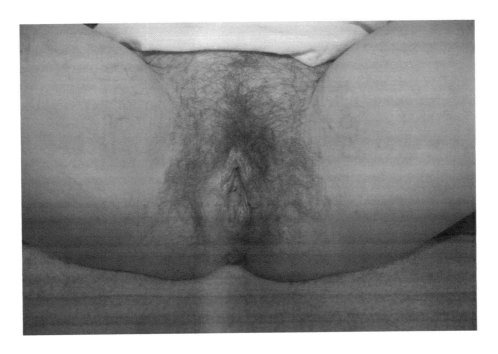

> Join the Revolution: *Let Your Vagina Breathe!*
>
> Wear breathable fabric like cotton underwear—always. Do not wear underwear to sleep. Wear pantiliners only on special occasions like when your menstrual flow is light or right after sex so that semen and/or vaginal lubrication don't soak your underwear. Or maybe on days when your cervical fluid is really flowing and getting your underwear more wet than normal. But for anything short of this, join the revolution and don't wear pantiliners. A healthy environment for your vagina is one with lots of air, low moisture, and nothing to trap the moisture near or irritate the labia.

Suggested Resources:

Northrup, Christine. *Women's Bodies, Women's Wisdom: Creating Physical and Emotional Health and Healing* (New York: Bantam, 2010).

Raj, Roshini with Lisa Lombardi. *What the Yuck?: The Freaky and Fabulous Truth About Your Body* (Birmingham, AL: Oxmoor House, 2010).

Weschler, Toni. *Taking Charge of Your Fertility: The Definitive Guide to Natural Birth Control and Pregnancy* (New York: Harper Perennial, 1995).

I am forever indebted to this book. I read it when I was thirty-one years old and trying to get pregnant. I had been told all my adult life that I had polycystic ovarian syndrome, and I would have a difficult time getting pregnant. As soon as Marc and I decided we wanted to have a baby, I started reading books on fertility. I was absolutely amazed at what I did not know. I kept on thinking, as I read about cervical fluid and ovulation, that even though I had come so far — I had an undergraduate degree in psychology, a masters in public policy, I was well-read, open to new ideas — there was so much about my own body and my own vagina that I did not know. This thought marinated for many years and after having three children and hearing so many questions from my own daughter, I decided to write a book to try to address the fact that so many educated women really know so little about our own bodies.

CHAPTER 7

The Clitoris

LL: I was *wondering* why we didn't talk about the clitoris in the Rest of the Anatomy section. Now I see that it gets its very own section!

CG: Check out this montage of four pictures. In all four you can see a woman's clitoris, though the picture in the upper right is taken from a different angle than the other three. This is a picture of a fifty-seven-year-old lifting up the *clitoral hood* of her vulva to reveal the *glans clitoris*, a.k.a. clitoris. (Some people shorten this to *clit*, but I really don't feel comfortable with that. Just my personal quirk. But I think that many women, especially the younger generations, use that word more widely.)

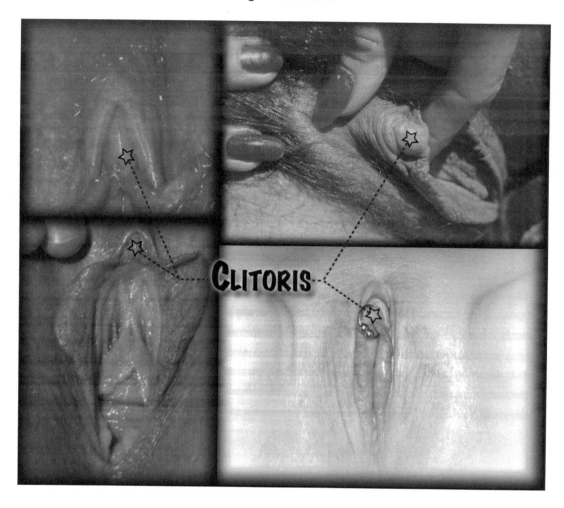

Anyway the glans clitoris is the most sensitive structure in the genital erogenous zone and the center of genital sexual pleasure in women. It is fairly small, about the size of a pencil eraser, though when aroused it can double in size.

The clitoris (you've probably heard it pronounced cli-TOR-is or CLIT-or-is, and either way is right) is actually more than meets the eye. The glans clitoris is the part that you can see and touch. But the glans clitoris is also attached to a firm yet rubbery and movable shaft that is approximately an inch long and connected to the pubic bone. The shaft divides and spreads to form roots (crura) that also attach to the pubic bone. You can't see any of this — it is all under some muscle and the mons. You can only see the eraser-sized clitoris. Here is a diagram where you can see all of the different parts, most of which are under the surface:

The Clitoris

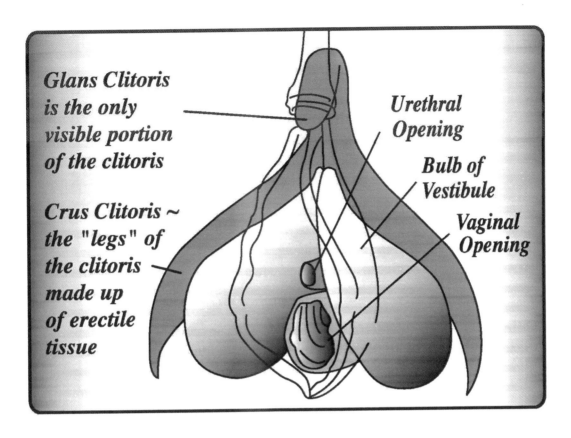

The most fascinating thing about the clitoris is that it is the only part of the human body—male or female—that has the *sole* purpose of pleasure. It does not serve any other purpose.

LL: What about a man's penis?

CG: Of course that gives him pleasure, but penises are also responsible for depositing semen into the vagina to make babies and for helping men urinate. Women have separate body parts to urinate and to make babies. But the clitoris is a world unto its own. A clitoris has thousands of nerve endings—double the number of nerve endings in the penis, by the way. The clitoris has approximately 8,000 nerve endings compared to 4,000 in the penis.

LL: Lucky us!

CG: Because there are so many nerve endings in a woman's clitoris, most women do not like direct stimulation to the clitoris. Rather, most women prefer indirect stimulation—stimulation to the shaft or the whole mons, the perineum or the labia. This stimulates the clitoris without making it feel too sensitive like when it is being touched directly.

Most experts agree that no matter how an orgasm happens, whether through someone's hands or penis or vibrator or tongue, female orgasm always results from some kind of clitoral stimulation.[25]

LL: What about reproduction? Doesn't the clitoris serve a purpose in reproduction? Couldn't you argue that since it feels good, more women will want to have sex, and that leads to more procreation?

CG: There is a definite argument there, but women can still procreate without a clitoris. At the 2002 conference for Canadian Society of Women in Philosophy, Dr. Nancy Tuana asserted that the clitoris is unnecessary in reproduction, but that this is why it has been "historically ignored," mainly because of "a fear of pleasure. It is pleasure separated from reproduction. That's the fear." She reasoned that this fear is the cause of the ignorance that veils female sexuality.[26]

LL: Does the clitoris remain sensitive throughout a woman's lifetime?

CG: That is a good question. No, on average the amount of sensitivity decreases over time. Just like our sense of smell and sight lessens over time so does our clitoral sensitivity. As women get older they may like direct stimulation more, and they may need more of this to have an orgasm.

LL: That's it? You are done with this section?

CG: Short and sweet — just like the clitoris!

Join the Revolution: *Fully Embrace the Fact That Vaginas Are For Pleasure!*

Yes, they can be for procreation, too. But the clitoris is the *only* human (male or female) body part whose *sole* purpose is for pleasure. The only conclusion we can draw from that is that God or Mother Nature or the Universe *wants* women to experience and seek out pleasure. Caveat: always practicing safe sex can ensure that the pleasure can continue…

---

25 W.D. Petok, "A Practical Approach to Evaluating Female Sexual Dysfunction," *ObG Management* (1999 Mar): 68 cited in Elizabeth Stewart, *V Book: A Doctor's Guide to Complete Vulvovaginal Health*, (New York: Bantam, 2002), 116.
26 Richard Cairney, "Exploring Female Sexuality," *ExpressNews* October 21, 2002, accessed December 21, 2011, http://liveweb.archive.org/http://www.archives.expressnews.ualberta.ca/article/2002/10/3201.html.

Suggested Resources:

Dweck, Alyssa and Robin Westen. *V Is For Vagina: You're A-to-Z Guide to Periods, Piercings, Pleasures and So Much More*, (Berkeley, CA: Ulysses Press, 2012).

Herbenick, Debby. *Because It Feels Good: A Woman's Guide to Sexual Pleasure and Satisfaction* (Emmaus, PA: Rodale Books, 2009).

Livoti, Carol and Elizabeth Topp. Vaginas: An Owner's Manual (Cambridge, MA: Da Capo Press, 2004).

CHAPTER 8

The Look of a Vagina

LL: It has been interesting seeing the differences in the look of the vaginas in earlier chapters in the book. Maybe I sneaked too many peeks at the *Playboy* and *Penthouse* magazines my older brother had hidden under his bed in his room when I was younger, but the vaginas in these pictures are a lot different from those vaginas in the magazines.

CG: Well, that's just like comparing your body to the bodies in *Vogue* and *Glamour* and all those other fashion magazines. If you compare yourself to *someone else's idea* of perfection, you will never be happy. Besides, most of those pictures are totally Photoshopped, and the graphic artists make the women's bodies look even better than they actually do.

LL: I don't think they had Photoshop in those days.

CG: Ha! You're right. It was airbrushing back then. But I can promise you, from working with vaginas for a living that I have never seen a real woman with a vagina that looked like one of the vaginas in those magazines.

Now look back at the montage of pictures in chapter 4 and tell me what races and weights these women are...and if they have had vaginal deliveries or not.

LL: It's really hard to tell because the pictures are so close up.

CG: True. The point I want to make here is that vaginas are like ears or faces — they are all different and all normal. Sometimes they look slightly different depending on the amount of fatty tissue (this tends to decrease as women get older, as does the natural lubrication and stretchiness), the pigment, the size of the vaginal opening, and the size and shape of the labia.

LL: It is very difficult for me to see the nuances.

CG: The vaginal opening will vary in size, and the hymenal remnants are difficult to see. Labia are generally uneven, and there is much to assess. I can tell approximately how old a woman is by looking at her vagina. I can mostly tell by how plump it is — this is caused by the amount of estrogen in the vagina. You probably cannot tell because this is not your line of work.

The one thing that you *can* notice, and something many people have strong opinions about, is a woman's choice of whether or not she shaves or waxes her pubic hair.

TO SHAVE OR NOT TO SHAVE

LL: Yes, we women spend so much of our lives shaving our legs, stressing about getting that bikini wax before that trip to the beach, and wondering if our vaginas look good or if we should be shaving them or doing something differently.

Why do so many people care? Not that I am exempt here. I have absolutely been influenced by society when it comes to obsessing over pubic hair. But why? When I think about it, and I am not in that moment getting ready to go to the pool, then all the concern about it just does not make sense to me. *Plus* I feel like I have spent so much *money* on trying to get rid of hair.

The Look of a Vagina

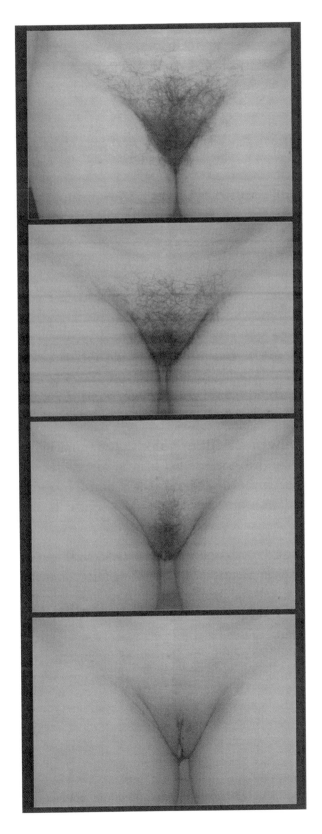

CG: It is definitely something that women obsess about, or if not obsess, at least spend a lot of time and energy thinking about. For example, you probably didn't realize how many different ways one could categorize pubic hairstyle—but check this out:

> *Different Styles of Pubic Hair*
>
> <u>Natural</u> (also called Au Naturel and Bush) is where nothing is done at all and the growth occurs naturally.
>
> <u>Trimmed</u> is where the pubic hair is trimmed with scissors so that the "bush" is smaller and neater.
>
> <u>Landing Strip</u> is where the hair is shaved or waxed on both sides so that what remains is one thick or thin line.
>
> <u>Partial Brazilian</u> is where the pubic hair is completely removed, except for a small remnant of very short hair right above the vulva.
>
> <u>Full Brazilian</u> (also called Hollywood) is when all the pubic hair is removed.
>
> <u>Patterns</u> is where the pubic hair is sometimes shaved or cut or waxed to create a pattern like an arrow, a heart, spade, small triangle, or pyramid, or whatever else strikes someone's fancy!

LL: What percent of women *shave*? How do they shave? I am so curious!

CG: I only see a small percent of the population in Charlotte, North Carolina. For a more national answer to this question, I went back to the survey by Harris that was commissioned by Vagisil.[27]

---

[27] Armen Hareyan, "New Survey Reveals Women's Attitudes About Feminine Health," April 5, 2006 http://www.emaxhealth.com/4/5373.html.

The Look of a Vagina

> The Vagisil survey found that:
>
> **One-fourth (25 percent) of all women aged eighteen and older report that they "closely trim their pubic hair with scissors or clippers."
>
> **Almost one-fourth (23 percent) say they shave part of their pubic hair off.
>
> **Nine percent say they shave all of their pubic hair off.

The survey goes on to report that women aged eighteen to forty-four are more likely to remove hair in their pubic region than women over forty-five, perhaps because this age group is more likely to think that men prefer a well-manicured pubic region on a woman.[28]

Pubic hair preferences are definitely generational. In the late ninties, shaving and waxing were not expected, but by two thousand five or so they were more or less expected in the younger generations. Perhaps this is because of what women and men saw in pornography.

Also, pubic hair is a *socially normed* thing in the same way that hairstyles are. In other words some styles are in and others are out. (Remember the Farrah Fawcett? Or the Dorothy Hamill? Or more recently the Rachel?) So there's not a right or wrong—it's all about what styles are popular, what styles work best for you, and so on.

The downside of things that are socially normed is that when you do something to be in style, it may not feel right for you. One example is if all your friends shave their pubic hair or get Brazilians, and you would prefer to go natural but get waxed anyway to fit in. That is not being true to who you are and what you like. Plus, to add insult to injury, I have some patients who complain of ingrown hairs, irritation, and even infection from grooming. One in six women (seventeen percent) experiences itching or irritation following pubic hair removal.

You've got to remember, too, that some people naturally have more hair than others. For example, Asian women, like Asian men, generally don't have a lot

---

[28] Thirty-eight percent of women aged eighteen to forty-four think most men prefer a manicured look, compared to 14 percent of women aged forty-five to fifty-four and 3 percent of those aged fifty-five and older.

of body hair. Women from Greece or the Middle East and similar places tend to have dark, coarse hair that is very noticeable. African American women have dark, curly hair, but it can blend with their skin tone. Scandinavian women, or any women who are naturally blonde, have naturally light pubic and body hair. And usually, a woman who chooses to do something drastic like getting a Brazilian is a woman with dark, coarse hair. This procedure tends to cause irritation and ingrown hairs.

LL: I'm one of those people who has dark, coarse hair…and pasty white skin… so my hair has always been so noticeable. But I just hate shaving—under my arms, my legs, pubic hair—I don't care. I just hate shaving. For most of my life I avoided shaving at all costs. When I do shave, I get ingrown hairs, and it is so painful and uncomfortable.

CG: Does this cause any kind of problem? For example, does your husband care if you shave?

LL: I don't think so. I've never asked. He just knows I hate shaving. However, my lack of shaving does bother one person—my mother! For my entire life (well, since puberty), my mom has always tried to get me to shave more. You know how moms are, trying to improve you and make you more attractive. She has given me so many razors and so much shaving cream over the years, and it all just sits unused in my bathroom! So, last year she gave me the gift of laser hair removal. I thought I would get it done just to get her to stop bugging me about not shaving my legs and so on. I got my lower legs, underarms, and bikini area done.

CG: Ouch.

LL: Ouch is right—it was painful! You're supposed to go about seven times or so to get all the hair to go away—the lasers literally burn and kill the hair follicles so they don't grow any more. I made it six times for my lower legs, and I only have a few random hairs growing now. But I only lasted through three laser treatments for my underarms and bikini area because it was just so painful. On the upside, it has really thinned out my hair, and I actually do like it better.

CG: Doesn't it hurt less each time you go? After they kill the hair follicles, don't they have fewer follicles to kill next time?

LL: I thought that would be the case, but it hurt just as much each time. I tried all those special creams and stuff to help, but it was still way too painful. But for some reason my lower legs didn't hurt as much, so it was more tolerable, and I had much more success with the hair removal. I might just go back to electrolysis—which also hurts, but much less. With electrolysis they only remove one hair at a time, and you have to go back a few times to get rid of some hairs. But it makes it easy to target that one annoying hair on your lip or toe or nipple. Overall I like that method better, if I have to choose any method of hair removal. But I have friends who prefer laser hair removal so to each her own.

Can you please end with a few interesting facts about pubic hair? You know, maybe for some good cocktail party conversation…or at least book club conversation.

CG: OK, here is one—do you know what the purpose of pubic hair is? Pubic hair actually has a role in attraction. Pheromones are trapped on your pubic hair and even if you wash your skin, your scent lingers in your hair. Both men and women give off pheromones—a smell that we cannot consciously identify but can detect at a subconscious level. Women, on average, end up picking partners to mate with who will produce healthier offspring. A woman can detect the difference between men who will make good babies with her and ones who will not, and she will consider the former more attractive. It is truly fascinating.[29]

Two—children do not have pubic hair, but as they get ready for puberty, they start to get soft, fine hair on their genitals. As puberty begins, the body produces more sex hormones, called androgens that cause the hair to go from being soft to darker, curlier, and coarser. The changes happen quickly, though the amount of skin covered with this hair changes and increases at a slow rate over a few years.

Three—pubic hair and armpit hair can be a different color than the hair on your head! It is usually darker, but in some people it is lighter. It is usually closest to the color of your eyebrows.

LL: So interesting. Thank you!

Suggested Resources:

O'Brian, Douglas. *101 Gynecology Views: 101 Open Vaginas*. Charleston, SC: CreateSpace, 2010.

---

[29] Jelto Drenth, *The Origin of the World: Science and Fiction of the Vagina* (London: Reaktion, 2004), 242-246.

O'Brian's book is a book of 101 pictures of vaginas—there is no text! But it is fascinating to look at the variety of shapes, colors, and angles. I did try to get in touch with Douglas O'Brian, but despite all of my detective skills, I could not find him anywhere. I wondered to myself if he created this book more for porn than for health education, but the truth is I see it much more as the latter.

CHAPTER 9

Smell

CG: As we have already mentioned tangentially, vaginas have a natural scent. Some women's vaginas smell more strongly, and others rarely give off any smell. With most women, the scent changes depending on the time of the month.

In a natural cycle, a woman gives off the strongest vaginal smell in the days between menstruation and ovulation, due, it is thought, to the hormonal condition of the vaginal wall.

Men have odors, too, and some men produce fatty acids just like some women do.

LL: Out of curiosity, I went online and did a search for vagina and smell, and I found a great discussion on a website called pheromonetalk.com. One person had asked others to try to describe the smell of a healthy vagina so he could try to replicate it in a pheromone product he was making. Participants had all kinds of descriptive responses. Here are a few[30].

> "Pungent, musky, damp, but not foul…earthy undertones…sort of like your body odor—some days stronger than other days…fruity (melon, soft-fleshed tropical fruits) with a slight tang, more mellow-sweet… oceanic (salty, fresh/amine—this part is very subtle)…Floral (again, very subtle: think hawthorn, acacia, meadow florals like yarrow, slight jasmine—very slight trace of indole—other copulins have overdone the indole, though)…a light jasmine scent, with added musky odors…sweet, light, salty, buttery, musk with high back palate tone of citrusy melon… but more complex than that. Hits your palate like butterscotch…add just a touch of copper to that…it smells like the ocean, fresh seafood—FRESH, not stinky old seafood—and sometimes it has a spicy aroma too…you know how absolutely soft and salty the freshest of shrimp smells?…Sweet comes to mind, but not candy sweet, more of a pungent fruit sweet. Fresh, clean comes to mind. A gentle muskiness, if that makes sense to you…"

CG: That is very interesting. Like lots of things in the human body, vaginas are affected by what you eat, where you are in your menstrual cycle, whether you have gone through menopause or not, what soap you use and many other factors. I have also heard that vegetarians tend to have a lighter vaginal smell.

LL: You mentioned that the smell is stronger between menstruation and ovulation. I take it that there is a cycle to the odor, just like there is a cycle to the bleeding?

CG: Yes. It is all interrelated. The smell follows the same cycle of the hormones that also cause you to ovulate and menstruate. But when you smell something that is *unusual for you* or if the smell does not change with the normal cyclical changes, then **definitely go see your doctor.**

LL: Why do you think so many women are uncomfortable with the smell of their vaginas, especially after hearing about all of those positive descriptors above?

---

[30] "What Does Your Healthy Vagina Smell Like While Ovulating?" *PheroTalk*, accessed June 2012, http://www.pheromonetalk.com/womens-pheromone-advice-tips-tricks/copulin-research-what-does-your-healthy-25035.html.

Smell

CG: Unfortunately, many, many women are uncomfortable with the smell of their vaginas. Almost one in four women (23 percent) indicate that they are "very conscious" of their vaginal or external vaginal odor, with one in six (17 percent) saying that they are self-conscious about it when being intimate with a partner. Ten percent of women take that a step further and report using products to combat vaginal odor.[31]

The survey also goes on to report that almost half of U.S. women (47 percent) indicate that they use feminine health products for various purposes. Almost one in four (24 percent) women use feminine health products to clean the feminine area or to absorb excess discharge. Of those, the most common products used (by 12 percent) are feminine cleansing cloths.

Jelto Drenth's book *The Origin of the World: Science and Fiction of the Vagina*[32] explains the very complicated reasons why vaginas smell the way they do. I will try to simplify it.

> The group of substances in a woman's vagina that are responsible for the fishy odor are called *amines*. They are produced by the breakdown of proteins. In animals, these short-chain volatile fatty acids (chemicals) are called copulins [like copulate] because the presence or absence of these signals determines whether or not the female is sexually attractive to the male! A majority of women—two thirds—only secrete other kinds of acids from their vaginas, so their odor may be called neutral. The other third of women produce fatty acids, and when those break down, they break down into proteins and amines, and that is what tends to smell.[33]

Join the Revolution: *Embrace the Smell of Your Vagina!*

What woman has not worried at least once in her life about how her vagina smells? Any OB/GYN will tell you that *most* of the time *most* women have very "normal"-smelling vaginas. Yet there are the facts and then the fear—the fear of someone else smelling your vagina!

---

31 Hareyan, "New Survey Reveals Women's Attitudes About Feminine Health."
32 Drenth, *The Origin of the World: Science and Fiction of the Vagina*, 240–241.
33 Bonsall and Michael, 1978.

> In short, every woman has a good handle on how her vagina smells. Unless you notice a very unusual smell—which could be a symptom of an infection—your normal smell is very likely a natural scent that does not need to be covered up.
>
> In a recent poll, about one-quarter of women in North America indicated that they don't like the smell of their vagina. You know what? Vaginas smell like vaginas! Half the women in the world have a noticeable vaginal smell—though some are stronger than others, and almost all women have vaginas that smell differently at different times of their menstrual cycles or stages in their lives.

LL: I wish that women felt more comfortable with their smell. I tried to bring up the topic with my female colleagues when I worked at a different school, and the conversation morphed into how often we all washed our pants—which is definitely relevant to the subject, but not exactly what I was getting at!

CG: So what was the consensus?

LL: Well, this was a very unscientific sample of about ten middle school teachers, counselors, and secretaries, and the conversation went on throughout the day during class changes and lunch and so on. But I would say the consensus was that most women wore their pants for three days before washing them. One woman dry-cleaned everything every time she wore it, but she was definitely the exception to the rule.

I do wish that women in general would feel more comfortable with the smell of their vaginas. I worry about the health of vaginas when we put harsh chemicals on them. Vaginas are a mucous membrane and can absorb these chemicals. Many OB/GYNs I interviewed for this book were very much against women putting harsh chemicals on or around vaginas. One went as far as to say that vaginas are like rain forests and we would never want to throw chemicals into a rain forest. But I also understand that every woman is different and every woman balances things in her own way

CG: Here are some things to consider for any woman who has this issue.

If you have a vaginal odor you don't like:

1. Be sure to shower or bathe regularly. But do not use harsh chemicals on your vulva. Use mild soap or just warm water, and wash between all the creases with your fingers. Be sure to let the warm water run over your vulva. If you use a washcloth, make sure to use a newly washed one each time because wet sponges and washcloths lying around the shower create a good environment for bacteria to grow.

2. Are you wearing all-cotton underwear that fully covers your vulva? Thongs and other smaller underwear may not absorb your natural vaginal discharge (and they may also irritate the skin). One OB/GYN friend of mine says that thongs are like a "tightrope for bacteria" to walk from the anus to the vagina. When bacteria grow in vaginas, they can cause an unpleasant smell.

3. Are you sure the self-consciousness is not just that—self-consciousness? Can you ask a close friend or partner, if they smell anything? If they do not, then perhaps you are being too sensitive about this natural smell.

4. Is the odor on your *vagina* or on your *clothes*? If it is on your clothes, try washing your clothes more frequently.

5. Some fabrics pick up and actually exacerbate vaginal odor. Exercise clothes, synthetic materials, and pantyhose are all examples of this. If you have clothes that exacerbate vaginal odor, it might be a good idea to get rid of them and opt for more natural fabrics.

6. Consider spraying perfume on your stomach or legs, but not directly on your vulva because this could be an irritant.

7. Consult with a doctor to rule out potentially more serious problems like bacterial vaginosis (BV) or sexually transmitted infections (STIs—see appendix 3).

8. If you have tried all of this (including going to the doctor) and you are still aware of an odor that is abnormal, then ask your doctor

> for some suggestions. If she does not have any suggestions, consider consulting with another doctor who may. If you feel like you need to use a product to cover up the smell, then use it with extreme caution. Be cautious about applying chemicals, fragrances and soaps to your vulva. There are products by Vagisil and other companies that cover up some of the odor, but we suggest using them as a last resort.

I am going to conclude with a quote from Eve Ensler of *The Vagina Monologues* fame.

LL: She is my idol! An absolute living goddess. *Vagina Revolution* definitely stands on the shoulders of *The Vagina Monologues,* and if I had not seen that show in Charlotte many years ago, I probably would not feel as comfortable as I do discussing these topics we've been discussing. Not that I am one hundred percent comfortable yet, but I am so much closer than I've ever been. So I thank Eve Ensler for being part of my own personal evolution.

CG: I am so with you. She is an amazing soul.

LL: And she started V-Day, which has been advocating an end to violence against women and girls worldwide. See http://www.vday.org/home_for more information.

CG: So let's conclude this section with her wise words:

> My vagina doesn't need to be cleaned up. It smells good already. Don't try to decorate. Don't believe him when he tells you it smells like rose petals when it's supposed to smell like pussy. That's what they're doing—trying to clean it up, make it smell like bathroom spray or a garden. All those douche sprays—floral, berry, rain. I don't want my pussy to smell like rain. All cleaned up like washing a fish after you cook it. I want to taste the fish. That's why I ordered it.[34]

Suggested Resources:

Ensler, Eve. *The Vagina Monologues.* New York: Random House, 2007.

Drenth, Jelto. *The Origin of the World: Science and Fiction of the Vagina.* London: Reaktion, 2004.

---

34 Eve Ensler, *The Vagina Monologues* (New York: Random House, 2007).

CHAPTER 10

Feel

LL: This is a weird question. How would you say a vagina is supposed to feel?

CG: I know it sounds strange, but basically if you don't think about how your vagina is feeling at any given time, then you probably don't have anything you really need to worry about.

It's when you *do* think about how your vagina is feeling—like having the symptoms of a yeast infection or a urinary tract infection—then you might need to worry. For example, if you feel any kind of pain or itching, you should see your doctor to find out the cause.

But with a normal vagina you should feel nothing. Your vulva should be soft and pliable. I would almost describe it as dewy. It should not be dry, rather it should be a bit moist. It should be pain free and not itchy. The inside of your vagina should be a bit wavy from the rugae, and it should be full and plump. It's a mucus membrane, like the inside of your mouth, and all mucus membranes are meant to be moist. The mouth has salivary glands to keep it moist, and the vagina has lubricating glands as well.

Sometimes your vagina will feel more lubricated than usual. For example when you are sexually aroused or having intercourse the vaginal tissue will become fluffy and puffy and brighter red. This change actually prepares the vaginal tissue for penetration.

Speaking of intercourse, penetration should not hurt. Your vagina is designed for intercourse, and it has the perfect amount of space. The muscles at the opening of the vagina should be relaxed enough to allow for penetration. Sometimes some women need lubrication, especially for the initial penetration. Many women do not need this, and usually if a woman spends enough time in foreplay before penetration, she does not need any additional lubrication.

LL: So what happens if you are reading this and thinking *my vagina doesn't feel like this…I have itching or pain on the outside…or painful intercourse…or pain during other times and not just intercourse…?*

Itching and Pain

CG: In those cases a woman should see a health care professional because there are certain things she would want to rule out.

Itching and pain are both very common. Remember that same study I cited in the section on smell, the one conducted by Harris Interactive for Vagisil? That study found that forty-three percent of U.S. women aged eighteen and older indicated that they had experienced vaginal itching.[35] As for pain, pain may be felt in the vagina, deep inside the pelvis, or at the opening of the vagina. Sensations of pain can range from dull to throbbing to a burning or tenderness of the skin. Some women experience pain during intercourse, others after intercourse, and others experience pain when they are not having intercourse. According to the Association of Reproductive Health Professionals, fifteen percent of women at

---

35 Hareyan, "New Survey Reveals Women's Attitudes About Femine Health.

any given time report that they are experiencing painful intercourse. The medical name for this is dyspareunia.[36]

Here is another pain statistic that is worrisome to me—according to a survey by Brigham and Women's Hospital in Boston, Massachusetts, approximately sixteen percent of women between the ages of 18-64 have experienced chronic vulvar pain for at least three months or more.[37] The medical name for this pain disorder is vulvodynia. Its cause is not yet well understood. Some women suffer for months or even years with this.

There is some itching and some pain that can be easily diagnosed and taken care of. But there is other itching and pain that is more difficult to figure out. Like I said, some women spend months or even years trying to address a certain kind of itch or pain. Not all health care professionals know all the relevant questions to ask, and some health care professionals are better *medical detectives* than others.

There are many different kinds of health care professionals who can help with issues involving a woman's vagina. I will only name a handful, but I am also going to illustrate this with a Venn diagram to visually show that not all medical professionals can help you with every condition you may experience. This is why it is important to remember that **if you have chronic pain or itching and you have concluded in any way that you should *just live with it* or it is *normal*, you are wrong!** By the way, you are not alone. How many women do you know who just tough it out or live with something that is not comfortable in some way?

LL: Every woman?

CG: Exactly! But it should not be this way. Here are a few examples:

I had one patient who went to an OB/GYN about painful intercourse, and she was told to use more lubrication during intercourse. She lived like that for ten years until one day she overheard a few women speaking about a Vulvovaginal specialist. She made an appointment with that specialist and was diagnosed with something that was very rare but very curable.

I also have had many other women in similar predicaments who have gone to a physical therapist who helped strengthen or relax their pelvic floors. Physical therapy on your pelvic floor can do all kinds of wonders.

---

36 Good In Bed website accessed November 2012, http://www.goodinbed.com/miniguides/2010/01/pain-during-vaginal-intercourse.php.

37 B. L. Harlow and E. G. Stewart, A Population-Based Assessment of Chronic Unexplained Vulvar Pain: Have We Underestimated the Prevalence of Vulvodynia? *JAMA* 58 (2003):82-8.

I have also had other women who have gone to their internists or family doctors with issues of incontinence, and the doctors have told them that this is something that comes with age. OK, maybe it does happen more frequently with age, but this does not mean that we all have to start wearing Depends at age 45! There are many things that different kinds of health care professionals can do to address all kinds of issues regarding women's vaginas. With strengthening and coordination exercises much incontinence can be reduced.

LL: I know that as a patient if I go to a doctor — especially an OB/GYN who is knowledgeable about vaginas — and she tells me something then I am very likely to take her word for face value. If she tells me something is normal like having a bit of incontinence after childbirth, then I am likely not going to follow this up with another doctor. But I have learned during the course of writing this book that different medical professionals have different sets of knowledge and I should never assume that any one doctor knows all medical information. I was surprised at how all of the doctors and medical professionals were so honest and forthcoming about this. For example one marriage and family counselor told me that she has very little knowledge about sexual dysfunction, and because this can sometimes be at the root of a couple's issues, she needs to refer some couples to a sex therapist who can help solve these kinds of problems. This same counselor told me that OB/GYNs often do not know good sex therapists to refer to. All of this was very confusing to me at first because I had assumed that doctors had a more macro-approach — and when they were unfamiliar with an issue in their field then they would know exactly what kind of medical professional would know and then they would refer.

CG: Being in the medical field I am very aware of our field's limitations but also know that many patients think this way — they assume that if one doctor does not have the answer then they know who will. It is actually not so easy. Look at this Venn diagram:

And sear this image into your brain so you can access it if anyone ever tells you that there is a condition that you must live with. You may go to your OB/GYN, and she may not find anything wrong but perhaps a physical therapist will know how to fix that very problem you are having. Or perhaps a physical therapist cannot find anything wrong but a sex therapist can help you get to the root of your issue. Different health care professionals, even if they are all excellent, are more familiar with different bodies of information. Although their specialties may overlap, not all professionals will be familiar with or able to help with all conditions. **But if you are having an issue and one health care professional cannot find the answer or tells you there is no answer, then it**

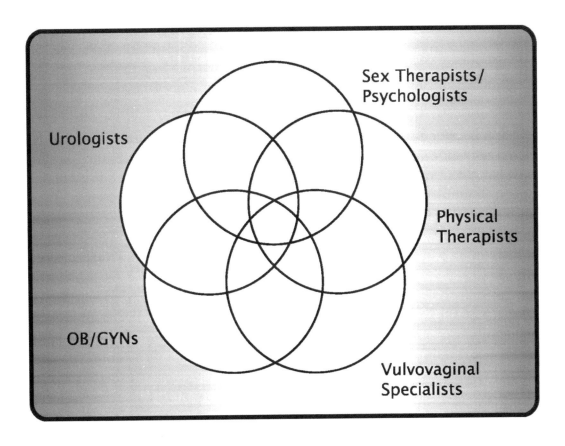

is your responsibility to keep trying to find the cause and the cure. You may have to refer yourself to other medical or psychological professionals. Now I also want to say that there is not a cure for everything. In some cases a patient may go to multiple health care professionals and never figure out the cause of her issue. But many women give up before trying different kinds of health care professionals. We are all way too willing to live with pain and discomfort.

LL: Do you think we should list some of the most common complaints women have? Or are there so many different conditions that we should just suggest that women see a health care professional?

CG: If a woman experiences itching on her vulva or in her vagina, she should see her doctor to rule out a long list of possible conditions and diseases. The most common are yeast infections, UTIs, and bacterial vaginosis, but there are also several skin diseases and conditions that are beyond the scope of this book, including eczema, lichen sclerosis, lichen planus, vestibulitis, or vulvodynia.

Over half of women who experience vaginal itching indicate that they will self-treat external vaginal itch or an infection with over-the-counter medications before going to the doctor. However, only thirteen percent indicate that they can always tell when external vaginal itch is the result of an infection. Personally, I am a big believer in sending women to the doctor if they have any unusual itching. The doctor can take a swab and look under the microscope to see if there is anything there they need to treat medically. If not, then there might be over-the-counter solutions.

When one of my patients has a complaint about an irritation, and it is not something that has the telltale signs of a yeast infection or a UTI, I sometimes suggest that she prevent any soaps, dyes, or chemicals from touching her vulva. She can try washing her underwear in a different detergent—one that is more natural or has no chemicals—and then not use any dryer sheets. She should try using different kinds of tampons or pads. Also, I always suggest that when washing your vulva in the shower, you should only use warm water and either very mild soap or no soap at all.

LL: Why no soap?

CG: Soap can be an irritant for some people. Not everyone. For thousands of years, women did not use soap, and we survived. I don't think it is necessary. I think if you take your fingers and run them over all the parts of your vulva while warm water is washing over you from the shower, that is just fine.

As for pain, if a woman experiences pain that lasts for more than a day, then she should see a doctor. Some pain is on the outside, like pain from the skin on her vulva or labia. Some women experience pain from their pelvic floor muscles, some pain could come from the bladder or from the uterus.

If a woman has occasional pain after intercourse or from wearing thongs and if resolves itself after a day or so, then it likely does not mean anything. But if a woman experiences persistent pain—anything that lasts more than a day, she should see a doctor.

Also, if a woman feels burning—again anything that lasts more than a day, she should see a doctor. This includes burning in her bladder, urethra, or vulva.

Dryness

CG: Many women experience dryness. Like I mentioned before, your vagina should be moist, but there are certain things that make a woman's vagina less moist. Some birth control pills can cause dryness. You may have to experiment with another kind of pill to see if this is the case. Other women have a condition where the glands that secrete lubrication stop working because of a disease or a blocked duct, just like you can have a blocked duct in your eye.

The most common causes of vaginal dryness are perimenopause and menopause. These are stages in a woman's life when she stops producing as much estrogen. We will have much more on this later in the book. As estrogen levels in your body decrease, so does lubrication to your vagina. One of the most common complaints about menopause is a woman says that her vagina feels dry. Although in general I don't think women should use chemicals anywhere near their mucus membranes, I make an exception for this. Vaginal dryness is really uncomfortable, and I would recommend using moisturizer on your vagina just like you do on your face if you have concluded that your vaginal dryness is due to perimenopause or menopause. In that case moisturizers are for daily use. Some women like products like Replens or Neogyn, and there are new products coming out all the time. If the idea of putting chemicals on your vagina bothers you, there are natural solutions such as olive oil and vitamin E caplets or roll-on. Any of these moisturizers should keep the tissue moist and more comfortable.

Some women feel they need to use a pantiliner to protect their underwear if they use moisturizer, but I would not recommend this. Wearing pantiliners absorbs moisture and causes even more dryness.

Maintaining sexual activity is a natural way to create a more lubricated and healthy vaginal environment.

LL: But if a woman already feels like her vagina is dry, then won't it feel worse to have sex?

CG: That is what lubricants are for. Lubricants, as opposed to moisturizers, are designed for intercourse. There are a lot of lubricants you can buy over the counter. My favorite one is Slippery Stuff because it doesn't contain propylene glycol, which is an alcohol and can sting the skin on some people's more delicate tissue. If a woman has sensitive skin then there are hypoallergenic lubricants. Many doctors suggest using KY Jelly, but it is very thick, so I suggest using a different kind of lubricant.

Issues of dryness during sex may be caused by some kind of sexual dysfunction or psychological feelings about sex. Sometimes it is difficult to determine if this is the case or not. If it is a possibility then it is very important to see a counselor and possibly get a referral to a sex therapist to examine what is going on. So often our health issues are directly related to our mental health issues.

Pelvic Floor Issues

CG: There are other things that women often feel in or surrounding their vagina, and there is a whole subsection of sensations that have to do with a woman's pelvic floor.

LL: Can you please explain what you mean by the pelvic floor? I want to make sure I have this straight.

CG: Sure. The pelvic floor muscles are sort of like a big hammock at the base of your pelvis. The pelvic floor consists of a deep muscle layer and a superficial muscle layer that support your pelvic organs (vagina, rectum, urethra, uterus).

Do you remember this image from chapter 3?

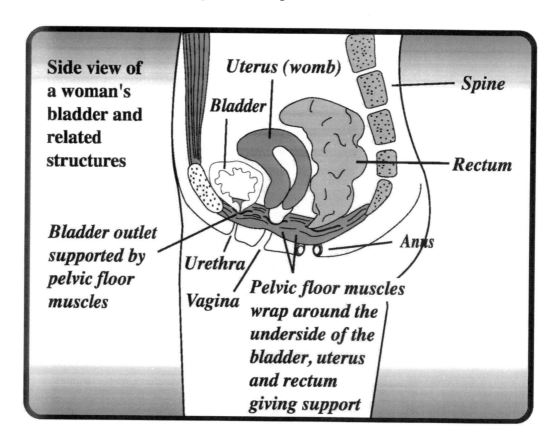

CG: The pelvic floor muscles form a figure eight, stretching between the pubic bone at the front and your coccyx or tailbone at the rear. An interesting aside here is that muscles are often named after the bones they are attached to so the muscle between the pubic bone and the coccyx bone is called the pubococcygeus or PC for short. The PC muscle is probably the best known muscle in the pelvic floor but it really only accounts for approximately one quarter of one layer of muscles in the pelvic floor. The urethra and vagina pass through the front hole of the figure eight and the rectum through the rear.

The muscles are usually tight and firm, but when they start to get weak you might notice some incontinence or other changes. When the muscles are too tight then you might notice that intercourse is painful or bowel movements can be painful or difficult. You can see the web of the pelvic floor muscles in the following diagram, and you can see the difference between tight muscles and weaker ones.

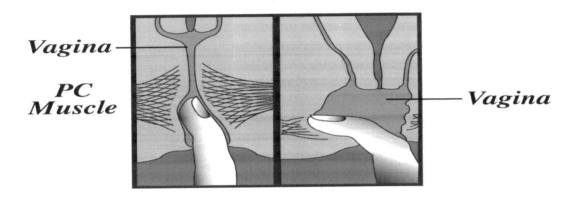

The PC muscles support the pelvic organs, bladder, and rectum, and their function is critical to activities such as urinating, having bowel movements, and sexual intercourse.

Exercises increase the blood flow to this region, which helps with healthy cell renewal, as well as adding strength and tone to the muscle itself. Like any other muscle, the PC muscles benefit from exercise and toning on a regular basis.

When the pelvic floor muscle weakens, a number of things can happen. A woman may develop urinary or stool incontinence, which is an inability to control the bladder or bowel. A weak pelvic floor muscle can also lead to poor muscle action during labor and delivery, a decrease in sexual pleasure, or genital prolapse, an uncomfortable condition in which the bladder, rectum, or uterus moves down into the vagina.[38]

---

38 "Where Are Your Pelvic Floor Muscles and Why Are They Important?" *My Pelvic Fitness*, accessed September 2012, http://www.mypelvicfitness.com/health.htm.

Something else important here is that pelvic floor pain is extremely common in women, and it is also debilitating. Approximately 15-20 percent of women experience some kind of pain of their pelvic floors at any one time, and approximately 25 million American women have experienced pelvic pain[39].

LL: What causes this pelvic pain?

CG: There is a wide range of things that cause either temporary or chronic (six months or longer) pelvic pain. A few causes include infection or inflammation; pain caused by the bowel, bladder or appendix; ectopic pregnancy; menstrual cramps; pelvic inflammatory disease (PID); ovarian cancer; ovarian cysts; kidney or bladder stones; vaginal infections; or vaginitis. The list goes on and on. I like how the Mayo Clinic sums it up, "Diseases and conditions of several body systems can cause pelvic pain, often as part of a group of symptoms that may not initially seem to be related to each other. Pelvic pain may arise from your lower intestinal tract, reproductive system, or urinary system. Pelvic pain may also arise from muscles, ligaments, or other pelvic floor tissues. Occasionally, pelvic pain may be caused by irritation of nerves in the pelvis.[40]"

LL: Wow—I never imagined that that one group of muscles could be influenced by so much!

CG: It is not just the muscle. There is so much going on in the whole region. I will try to get back to the topic at hand, vaginas, and also how pelvic floor pain and issues relate to vaginas.

I mentioned before that a lot of issues in the area are caused by a woman's pelvic floor being weakened. Sometimes this is due to childbirth, though not always. One of the miracles of a woman's body is that it is built to carry and deliver babies. But this can also often put a strain on a woman's body, and if she does not actively work to tone her pelvic floor muscles, they could get weaker.

LL: Is this sort of like doing Kegel exercises? I think all obstetricians prescribe them after their patients give birth. I know mine did.

---

[39] International Pelvic Pain Society, accessed November 2012, http://pelvicpain.org/news/eNews/september2012.pdf. If you are experiencing chronic pelvic pain, check out this patient information at http://pelvicpain.org/pdf/Patients/CPP_Pt_Ed_Booklet.pdf.
[40] Mayo Clinic, accessed November 2012, http://www.mayoclinic.com/health/pelvic-pain/MY00124/DSECTION=causes.

CG: Some women can improve the tone of their PC muscles by doing Kegel exercises. This is a kind of exercise that was named in the 1940s after Dr. Arnold Kegel.

LL: Wouldn't you just love to be a man and have your name remembered for all time by women squeezing their vaginal muscles?

CG: Ha! Kegel exercises are a great way to get your muscles back into shape, just as lifting weights can help your arms or legs.

LL: Ooh, I could use some of that.

CG: Couldn't we all! So many women care a lot about exercising to get their abs in shape or their arms or legs, but I rarely hear anyone express concern about getting her pelvic floor muscles in better shape[41]. Yet looking at that diagram you can see just how important the pelvic floor muscles are to your vagina, your urethra, your anus, and the whole region. **It is so important to keep your pelvic floor muscles toned and in good shape**.

Our bodies are such a miracle. The uterus is a muscle that is the size of a fist, but when we are pregnant our uterus expands to accommodate a baby. Our organs are all mobile and flexible. The uterus, the bladder, the rectum, and the intestines can all move over a bit to adjust to a pregnancy. And all those organs are supported by the pelvic floor muscles. We also have ligaments that attach to our organs that suspend them in the abdominal cavity. Our vagina is also supported by the pelvic floor muscles. There are muscles at the entrance of the vagina that relax and contract to make these accommodations. All of these muscles and organs are supported by the boney structures of the pelvis.

So all of that being said, we need to take good care of our pelvic floors. The best way to do that is to regularly exercise and tone our muscles. And how could we best do this? By doing Kegel exercises.

---

[41] As this book went into production I looked on the Vagina Revolution FaceBook page and heard from a woman in New Hampshire who runs a pelvic floor toning class at her yoga studio called Vagina Revolution—what a fabulous idea.

Kegel Exercises

<u>What</u>: Kegels are exercises that are designed to strengthen your pelvic floor muscles and keep them in shape.

<u>Why</u>: Your pelvic muscles support so many important organs, including your bladder, your uterus, and your bowels. By keeping your pelvic floor muscles in shape you can reduce many problems such as organ prolapse and incontinence. Strong pelvic muscles also help make recovery from childbirth easier. Other benefits include enhancing sexual pleasure because your vaginal muscles will be more toned.

<u>How:</u>

1. First identify your pelvic muscles. Know where your pelvic floor muscles are. You can feel them when you squeeze your muscles like you are trying to not pass gas. That is the feeling of squeezing your pelvic floor muscles. It's the muscle around your rectum, and it is also around your vagina and urethra. It even connects to your clitoris. If you squeeze really hard you can feel this. If you are not sure where the muscles are, here are two ways you can detect them:

    A. When you are urinating try to stop the flow of urine coming out of your urethra. Once you have identified that muscle don't do that any more. It's not a good idea to hold in your urine. But to identify your muscles then it is OK.

    B. A second way of finding your muscle is by putting your leg up on something, perhaps a stool or your toilet, and then inserting your finger into your vagina. Squeeze your muscles around your finger. If you can feel your vagina contracting, your pelvic muscles are in decent shape. If you don't feel anything or maybe just feel a small flutter, you absolutely need to do Kegel exercises.

2. Once you have identified the correct muscle, you are ready to begin the exercises. The exercise consists of squeezing and relaxing your muscle around your vagina, urethra and anus and then continuing to squeeze the muscles in your vagina. Use a

> squeeze-and-lift motion where you can almost feel the bottom of your abs tightening as well.
>
> 3. Squeeze your pelvic muscles and hold it for two seconds. Remember to squeeze in and then lift. Then relax for two seconds. It is just as important to relax as it is to squeeze. These two-second intervals are the short Kegels. You might not be able to squeeze for ten seconds yet, but with some practice you should be able to. Squeeze for ten seconds and then relax for ten seconds. These are the long Kegels.
>
> 4. Alternate between short and long Kegels. Start by doing Kegels for two to three minutes per day and work your way up to doing them for ten minutes per day.
>
> 5. Try to vary your position by doing exercises when you are lying down, sitting up, standing or even squatting. This way you will tone different parts of the muscle and you will train your muscles to operate in different positions.
>
> <u>When</u>: The good thing about Kegel exercises is that they can be done anywhere because no one can tell that you are doing the exercises. You can do Kegels while you are at work, in line at the grocery store, in your car, in a boring lecture or meeting, or trying to fall asleep at night.

LL: OK, so I have to admit I sort of let my doctor's advice go in one ear and out the other when she told me after my three vaginal births that I should do Kegel exercises. But now, eight years after my last child was born, I finally understand the importance and significance of doing Kegel exercises. I wish you had been there to tell me all of this after I had babies. I will definitely take these exercises more seriously now.

CG: You are not alone. Most OB/GYNs tell women to do these exercises when they go in for their six-week postbirth visits. But I don't think a lot of women take it seriously enough because they don't really understand the importance of keeping their pelvic floor muscles in good shape. If women don't keep their pelvic floor muscles in good shape, I may see them in my office again, either for prolapsed organs (when a bladder or vagina or rectum starts to *fall out*) or incontinence. Something I hear from patients after childbirth is the very common complaint about incontinence or leaking urine. A big complaint about vaginal delivery is that women have less control over holding their urine.

LL: Oh, baby, that has just been an ongoing problem for me since my first vaginal delivery. I thought that after my third delivery, it would get better. Wrong. I was walking with my friend Mara yesterday, and granted, I was holding in some pee, but *all of a sudden* I felt the urge to pee, and I did NOT make it to the bathroom. Luckily, she did not notice, nor did anyone else because we were doing a prework walk at six A.M., and no one was really around. But boy, was I happy to be close to a shower.

CG: Thank you for sharing!

LL: Hey, it's appropriate—we were talking about incontinence, right? It's not like incontinence is taboo or anything.

CG: Well, it does embarrass a lot of people. But it shouldn't. It is so unbelievably common. Stress incontinence affects one in three new mothers. And research shows that a lot of women are addressing the symptoms (the incontinence or leaking) and not the cause (the pelvic floor issues that may be going on). Research also shows that in the United States thirty-eight percent (4.5 million) of all menstrual pads sold are used to self-treat incontinence. And this issue is not just in the United States. Research further shows that 200 million people worldwide suffer from incontinence.[42]

LL: I heard you say stress incontinence, and I have heard before that there are different kinds of incontinence.

CG: First there is a difference between urinary incontinence and fecal incontinence. The former involves the urethra and leaking urine, and the latter involves the anus and rectum and leaking feces. I will concentrate on urinary incontinence. There are a few different kinds of urinary incontinence. But there are two main kinds:

Stress Incontinence

CG: Stress incontinence is when a woman (or man) involuntarily leaks urine. It is caused by *stress* on the bladder that is triggered by coughing, sneezing, laughing, exercising, or lifting. This kind of incontinence is the most common type of incontinence among women.

---

42 "Where Are Your Pelvic Floor Muscles and Why Are They Important?" *My Pelvic Fitness*, accessed September 2012, http://www.mypelvicfitness.com/health.htm.

Causes of stress incontinence include pregnancy and childbirth, which cause stretching and weakening of pelvic floor muscles. Causes also include a hormone imbalance or a decrease in estrogen following menopause, weakening in the wall between the bladder and the vagina, or a change in the position of the bladder. Other factors may also increase the risk for stress incontinence such as being overweight.

My favorite part of this talk about incontinence is treatment. To improve or eliminate incontinence, women can make lifestyle changes and/or get treatment, depending on which type of incontinence they have and what the cause is. Treatment includes pelvic floor exercises (Kegels), biofeedback, physical therapy, devices (such as a pessary that can be inserted into the vagina to support the organs and reduce leakage), injections, and in extreme cases surgery.

Urge Incontinence

CG: Urge incontinence is a sudden, strong urge to urinate, followed by an involuntary loss of urine. **Women should not have to urinate more than seven to nine times a day, and they should be able to sleep through the night without having to get up to urinate (at least until approximately age sixty), but women with urge incontinence may need to do both.** Also if a woman needs to urinate (or move her bowels), she should be able to drive home or finish what she is doing, walk to the restroom, and not have to rush to the toilet.

Causes of urge incontinence include age, damage to the bladder's nerves or surrounding muscles (sometimes because of an episiotomy or tear during childbirth), urinary infection in the bladder or kidneys, surgery, or other diseases or conditions.

Urge incontinence can be treated by timed voiding and bladder training, medications, electrical stimulation, and sometimes by surgery. Women can also decrease symptoms by reducing bladder irritants, including caffeine and soft drinks.

LL: What do you mean by bladder training?

CG: If a woman has urge incontinence, and she has ruled out the cause being a disease or infection, she should try to better control her urination. She can increase her voiding intervals to increase the amount of volume she could hold. If she has a sudden urge to urinate, she can distract herself and think about something else while calmly walking to the toilet. She should try counting to 20. In many cases over time she can retrain her bladder. She should also consume less caffeine. Caffeine is not good for urge incontinence. And definitely do pelvic floor exercises—a good squeeze for ten seconds and then relax for ten seconds for at least a few minutes a day. She should see some results in a few weeks.

There are other kinds of incontinence as well and some people experience two types of incontinence simultaneously—this is called mixed incontinence.

Also, some women have temporary incontinence. For example if they recently went through childbirth, but they are able to tone their pelvic floor muscles, then the incontinence may not last. Women can also experience incontinence that is caused by certain medications.

Prolapse

CG: In some cases, a woman loses her vaginal tissue strength following a normal birth delivery and has an increased risk of pelvic organ prolapse. Pelvic organ prolapse is when a pelvic organ, like your bladder, uterus, urethra, vagina, or rectum prolapses—or drops—from its normal spot. Remember the picture where all the organs are neatly stacked? Well if your pelvic floor gets weak or strained, those organs can fall. This usually happens as a result of childbirth or surgery. It can be very uncomfortable.

LL: Like the feeling of your uterus sort of falling out through…your vagina?

CG: Yes. Or any of those other organs falling through. In most cases, your organs don't completely fall through, but they can. In many women this is just temporary. The organs may fall or adjust a bit, but it does not get worse over time. But this is also something that does not tend to get better over time.

LL: What does it feel like? How do you know if you have some kind of organ prolapse?

CG: Often times a woman will say that she feels like something is falling out through her vagina or rectum. This may happen more when she is running, jumping, coughing, sneezing, lifting, or laughing. She might have a feeling of pressure from the pelvic organs pressing against the vaginal wall or maybe a feeling of fullness in her lower belly. It could also be a feeling of a pull or stretch in the groin area or even pain in the lower back. She may need to urinate a lot, or she may have pain in her vagina during sex. Or it might just be that she is constipated.

LL: It sounds like one of those things that is hard to diagnose. I mean, constipation—that could be caused by anything.

CG: Organ prolapse can be difficult to diagnose, but usually it is not. Most health care professionals, starting with your OB/GYN, can diagnose prolapse with a pelvic exam.

LL: Is there anything you can do to either prevent prolapse or if you feel one of your organs prolapsing, to help improve the situation?

CG: Yes. For one thing this is more common in women who are overweight. Losing weight is helpful. Also, we are back to Kegels again. Anything that can strengthen the muscles in your pelvic floor is helpful. And if a woman has a long-lasting cough or constipation, addressing those issues will help prolapse. Women should also avoid lifting heavy things because this puts additional strain on her pelvic floor muscles.

If the symptoms are bad, a doctor can have you fitted with a device called a pessary—just like we mentioned above when we were talking about incontinence. This device can actually hold an organ in place. It's removable, and you can actually adjust it yourself.

Another option is surgery, but that is the last option I recommend for *most* women. I usually only recommend surgery when a woman is finished having children, and she is experiencing pain as a result of the prolapsed organ or if the prolapse is causing her to not enjoy sex.

A Word About Childbirth

CG: We have been talking about a lot of the issues regarding the way our vaginas feel, and we have noted that in many cases these changes happen because of childbirth, in particular vaginal births. But I feel very strongly about pointing something out here. **Childbirth is one of the miracles of our body. Our bodies are designed to have babies. And a majority of women do have babies (approximately eighty percent). It is so natural and normal.**

The amount of stretchiness in the vaginal walls and muscles, like everything else, differs in different women. Some women have no problem delivering a baby. Their vaginal muscles relax to allow the baby to easily come down the birth canal and then the muscles start to tighten up again almost immediately and return to normal. They are usually not as tight as before, but, in most cases, there is not much damage.

In some women, however, vaginal delivery can cause muscle and pelvic floor damage. And if a baby is having a hard time coming out, and the doctor decides to make a cut—an episiotomy—to make more room for the baby to come out, that can occasionally cause some damage. Or if the woman has one or more vaginal tears, all of this could affect the vagina's healing after delivery.

But in most cases women are fine after delivery. I don't want to scare anyone about childbirth because it is such a normal, natural part of life, and most of the time the mother heals relatively quickly.

If a woman is experiencing pain or prolapse or something else, we have mentioned above after she delivers a baby, she should definitely see a health care provider. Sometimes she will tell you to do Kegels and wait to see what happens. Other times she will suggest physical therapy where a physical therapist can actually help you strengthen your pelvic floor, and in some cases she will recommend surgery. Remember that Venn diagram of different kinds of health care professionals? If you are not happy with the advice from one of the professionals, then absolutely see another. If you are experiencing pain, itching, dryness, prolapse, or anything else, you should NOT just be passive and live with it. You are the only one who knows how *you* feel, and if you feel like something is wrong, then it likely is. There are so many health care professionals out there who want to help you heal.

LL: You are so passionate about your work!

CG: I really am. I love helping patients, and I love when they heal.

Suggested Resources:

> Glazer, Howard I. and Gae Rodke, *The Vulvodynia Survival Guide: How to Overcome Painful Vaginal Symptoms and Enjoy an Active Lifestyle* (Oakland, CA: New Harbinger, 2002).

> Stewart, Elizabeth and Paula Spencer, *The V Book: A Doctor's Guide to Complete Vulvovaginal Health* (New York: Bantam, 2002).

CHAPTER 11

Your Vagina Over Time

LL: Phyllis Diller, one of the pioneers of American female stand-up comedy, once joked, "Maybe it's true that life begins at fifty…but everything else starts to wear out, fall out, or spread out."

And how about this one — this time from Mark Twain, "Age is an issue of mind over matter. If you don't mind, it doesn't matter."

CG: You should not be talking here. And certainly not joking about this. You young 'un. You are in your forties, and I am an entire generation older than you are. I really have not minded getting older. I like the first half of Diller's statement about life beginning at fifty. It really does. So much worry is lifted, including fear of pregnancy, and as we get older we tend to experience much less self-consciousness. I have found it much easier to say what I mean and be myself. I feel much more authentic and true to myself.

Yes, it does mean that my body is changing...I liked my tighter arm and leg muscles. My friends who are in my generation complain that their breasts are sagging. They love to joke that their breasts look like "rocks in socks...!" But I don't mind my body aging a bit. Now I really understand how sexuality is much more about my inner self than about my body parts. In spite of the things that do change like sagging breasts, arms, chin, and skin, we can still feel very sexy and connected.

LL: You just reminded me of something Kate said to me when I was putting her in bed the other night. We went through our usual bedtime routine, and I walked to the door to turn around to give her yet another hug and kiss—this time from the doorway. Then she asked me a question, so I must have put my arm up against the door frame or something. I was in my pajamas, and I was not wearing a bra. She said to me, "Mommy, do this for a minute with your arm," and I put my arm up against the door frame again like she indicated. And then she let out a big "Oooohhhhh! NOW I know why women wear bras!" Thanks, Kate!

CG: That's too funny. But I say, "So what if a woman's boobs are starting to sag, and she has extra skin over her stomach? They are badges of honor from aging and childbirth." It's all in the mindset.

But let's get into the real conversation here—not just your body, but your *vagina* over time!

LL: Great!

CG: I am going to walk you through what happens to a vagina over time, from puberty through menopause and beyond.

Prepubescent Vaginas
In general girls' vaginas are very sensitive and delicate. It is not until hormones start to change that our old friend estrogen kicks in to plump up the vagina and make it more resilient. When a girl is prepubescent, her hymen can protect her vagina from foreign objects, but after estrogen thickens the vaginal tissue, it really does not need the hymen any more for protection.

Going Through Puberty

Girls start going through puberty any time between ages eight and thirteen. A girl's pituitary gland will release special hormones that will target her two ovaries. Her ovaries hold eggs that she has had since before she was born. These special hormones will cause her ovaries to start to make estrogen and both hormones will also prepare her body to start her periods and become pregnant some day.

An increase in estrogen causes girls to grow hair under their arms and in their pubic area. Pubic hair starts off soft and downy but then becomes darker, thicker, and curlier. Estrogen also causes changes to the color and thickness of the labia, and vaginal discharge increases. The hymen is still there, but it is small and sometimes undetectable.

Girls usually get their periods two years after their breasts first begin to develop. Girls should be able to use tampons even if they still have a noticeable hymen and tampon usage should not cause any pain or discomfort. Girls should also be able to tolerate a speculum exam at this point if they need one, though they usually do not need one.

Once a girl goes through puberty she can become pregnant.

LL: The onset of puberty and first getting a period seems to be a hot button for many women. In writing this book many women confided in me stories about when they first got their periods. I was surprised about hearing that many women were not told about their periods so when they first got their period, it caused a great deal of angst and worry. I am glad that we live in a time that is much more open about such things. If parents don't tell their kids today about periods, at least they learn about it in school.

CG: I hear period stories all the time, too. If you think about it any kid would be scared if she didn't know to expect a period, and all of a sudden blood started to flow out of her vagina — that is so scary. I, too, think it is a generational thing, but if anyone is reading this book and has a young daughter please be sure to talk to her about getting her period as soon as you start to notice she is going through puberty (you will first see breast buds start, and you might also notice her shape changing, more hair growing under her arms and in her pubic area, and she may start getting body odor, too).

Adulthood

As women move out of their teens and into their twenties and thirties, their periods become much more regular, they grow full pubic hair, and their labia often changes color. They have normal discharge, and their vaginal tissue should lubricate well and be capable of handling intercourse as many times a day or week as desired.

After Childbirth

Vaginas change a great deal to accommodate babies, but they usually go back to their former shape and architecture. After a few weeks or months a woman's vagina should go back to normal. Her labia should stay closed, remain moist, and you should no longer see the hymen in most women. Sometimes there will be very light scars from an episiotomy or from tearing.

Occasionally there will be major changes in architecture, especially with some fast deliveries or prolonged stages of pushing, both of which are hard on the vagina. In some cases a pelvic organ may prolapse as a result. If this happens, a woman should be sure to see a health care professional.

Perimenopause and Menopause

LL: I recently saw a great documentary called *Hot Flash Havoc*, and it taught me so much about menopause. But I would still love for you to go through a detailed definition and explanation of perimenopause and menopause. I am getting signs that make me think it is right around the corner.

CG: Sure. OK, first a definition of perimenopause and menopause.

> "Perimenopause, also called the menopausal transition, is the interval in which a woman's body makes a natural shift from more-or-less regular cycles of ovulation and menstruation toward permanent infertility, or menopause.

> "Women start perimenopause at different ages. In your forties, or even as early as your thirties, you may start noticing the signs. Your periods may become irregular—longer, shorter, heavier or lighter, sometimes more and sometimes less than twenty-eight days apart. You may also experience menopause-like symptoms, such as hot flashes, sleep problems, and vaginal dryness. Treatments are available to help ease these symptoms.

"Once you've gone through twelve consecutive months without a menstrual period, you've officially reached menopause, and the perimenopause period is over."[43]

Menopause is the permanent end of menstruation and fertility, defined as occurring twelve months after your last menstrual period.[44]

Second. The average age of menopause.

The average age of menopause in the United States is fifty-one. "Women typically menstruate for the last time at about fifty years of age. A few stop menstruating as young as forty, and a very small percentage as late as sixty."[45] For a variety of genetic and environmental factors, in rural, developing countries the average of age of menopause is earlier — around age forty-three.

Your mother's — and even your grandmother's — age at menopause may give you a clue to your own. If your mother or grandmother had an early menopause, you're apt to follow suit. Likewise, if they didn't stop menstruating until their early to mid-fifties, you may gain a longer stretch of fertile years. But this isn't cast in stone. A special workshop on Stages of Reproductive Aging, hosted by the National Institutes of Health in 2001, noted that individual women may be born with "a highly variable number of oocytes [eggs]" and that the rate at which they lose eggs also varies greatly. So talk to Mom, but remember, biology isn't necessarily destiny."[46]

And third. Some typical symptoms of perimenopause and menopause.

This list is culled from what I have seen with my patients, as well as from WebMD[47] and a really great website called 34 Menopause Symptoms.[48] I am going to list the most common symptoms below and put the rest — the ones

---

[43] "Perimenopause," *Mayo Clinic Diseases and Conditions*, September 16, 2010, accessed September 2012, http://www.mayoclinic.com/health/perimenopause/DS00554.

[44] "Menopause," *Mayo Clinic Diseases and Conditions*, August 10, 2012, accessed September 2012, http://www.mayoclinic.com/health/menopause/DS00119.

[45] "Understanding Menopause: The Basics," *WebMD*, n.d., accessed July 2012, http://www.webmd.com/menopause/guide/understanding-menopause-basics.

[46] "When Fertility Ends: The Average Age of Menopause," *Conceive*, March 5, 2009, accessed July 2012, http://www.conceiveonline.com/articles/when-fertility-ends-average-age-menopause.

[47] "Understanding Menopause: The Basics," *WebMD*, n.d., accessed July 2012, http://www.webmd.com/menopause/guide/understanding-menopause-basics.

[48] "Thirty-Four Menopause Symptoms," n.d., accessed August 2012, http://www.34-menopause-symptoms.com/.

from the 34 Menopause Symptoms website—in an appendix in the back (see appendix 4).

Please note that only about seventy percent of women experience menopausal symptoms. Some just have some of these symptoms, a small percentage of women will experience many or all, and some lucky women may not experience any symptoms.

- About 75 percent of women have hot flashes. Nighttime hot flashes are more common and may result in chronic sleep deprivation.
- The loss of estrogen and testosterone following menopause can lead to changes in a woman's sexual drive and functioning. Menopausal and postmenopausal women may notice that they are not as easily aroused, and may be less sensitive to touching and stroking—which can result in decreased interest in sex.
- Mood changes aren't as well understood, but some women report an obvious change in mood, including depression, anxiety, or increased stress.
- Women may experience vaginal dryness, painful intercourse, and urinary symptoms. These symptoms can be temporary but often they are not. There are ways to manage vaginal dryness, for example with moisturizers for daily use and lubricants for intercourse.
- According to the National Sleep Foundation, sixty-one percent of women have sleep disturbances because of menopause[49]. This could be caused by night sweats or hot flashes, both of which are caused by shifting hormones.
- Menopause increases your risk of osteoporosis (thinning of the bones) and heart disease. Speak with your doctor about this because some women are at more risk than others.
- Although women can get bladder control problems at any age, it is more common during menopause.

As a woman gets older, her skin loses some elasticity and thickness. A woman's vagina also gets thinner, and this makes it more sensitive and tender to the touch. Doctor's describe this as vaginal atrophy. When I first heard this, I thought they were talking about muscles. But they are not—they are talking about the thinning of the skin of the vagina, both inside and outside. Sometimes it actually hurts when a man's penis or a vibrator enters a woman's vagina. And when sex hurts, a woman ceases to feel turned on because, well, it hurts.

---

49 "Menopause and Sleep," National Sleep Foundation, accessed December 2012, http://www.sleepfoundation.org/search/node/61%25%20menopausal%20women.

So your vagina is not getting the natural lubrication that often comes along with sex. In addition to this, the low estrogen levels cause the vagina to be less naturally lubricated and dryer. The change in hormones can also leave the vagina feeling itchy and burning, even without having sex. The tissue is much more delicate so it is easy to irritate it. It's not really the hormones that do this, but the hormones make you more sensitive — to intercourse, to pads, to soaps.

LL: How do you know at that point that the itching or burning is not a UTI or yeast infection or something else like that?

CG: A woman should definitely go to her doctor to get a pelvic exam and a urine sample to make sure. Just as we said earlier, women often are wrong at self-diagnosis and that can be dangerous.

And then while you are at the doctor (or better yet, make a separate appointment just for this) ask about estrogen therapy. This is not right for everyone. I know medical professionals who are opposed to estrogen and some who are advocates for estrogen. Most professionals decide on a patient-by-patient basis. Some women who have had cancer or who are prone to cancer should not take estrogen because estrogen can actually "feed" the cancer. But many, many women do really well with estrogen. I personally use the estrogen that can be inserted directly into my vagina, and it has really helped keep my vagina less dry and irritated, and has helped my sex life a great deal. Other women take estrogen in the form of a suppository or a cream or a ring that is inserted in their vagina that releases estrogen. I prefer the insert because it puts less estrogen in my blood and focuses it in my vagina, where I need it and want it. BUT...

LL: I know — consult your doctor.

CG: Exactly. Every woman is different. Consult your doctor. If you don't like the answer you get, there is nothing wrong with getting a second or third opinion. Women should not suffer with painful sex or with itching or irritation either.

Something else that works for many women is adding more lubrication like Slippery Stuff or Astroglide while having sex. Make sure your lubricant is water based and not petroleum based (like Vaseline). If you use condoms, the petroleum can break down the latex in the condoms.

Moisturizers can also be used during the course of a normal day or after a shower — just as a woman may moisturize her face and arms and legs, she could put some moisturizer on her vulva.

> ## *Moisturizers vs. Lubricants*
>
> When it comes to managing vaginal dryness a lot of women are confused about the difference between the use of moisturizers and lubricants. Lubricants are for intercourse if a woman does not naturally lubricate during intercourse. There are many different kinds of lubricants, including Astroglide, Slippery Stuff, and KY products (but KY *jelly* may be too thick—try something less heavy).
>
> Moisturizers, on the other hand, can either be used daily or several times a week. Just like moisturizers we use on our faces. If you didn't put moisturizer on your face or hands, they could feel rough. When some women go through menopause their vaginas lose moisture and feel dry, too. Some even describe their vaginas as feeling like "the desert." If your vagina feels dry, you can moisturize for health and comfort reasons. There are lots of products out there, and there are new ones being developed all the time. Some moisturizers include Replenz, Me Again, Very Private, Silk-E, and Neogyn. Some of these moisturizers have more chemicals than others, and some may feel better to some women than others. If a woman prefers to go the more natural way, she can also use olive oil or vitamin E oil.
>
> A woman needs to know her body. A woman with very sensitive skin needs to be extra careful with her vaginal and vulvar tissue. Some women can tolerate different chemicals and some women can't.

Lastly, be sure not to make matters worse by douching. Women should not douche at any age, but during perimenopause and menopause it can actually wash out the little natural lubrication that your vagina does produce. Also, especially after menopause, always be sure to keep hydrated by drinking lots of water.

It is important to take good care of your vagina during this phase of your life not only for your own comfort, but also to maintain sexuality. Not surprisingly some women have less interest in sex during this time because of the changes in hormones and vaginal tissue. But it does not have to be this way. Perimenopause and menopause can be considered a new beginning sexually speaking. I read something years ago in a book called *What Your Mother Never*

Told You About S-E-X by Hilda Hutcherson that stuck with me. It must have been that I was reading it around the same time as I was going through menopause. Anyway, this is what she said.

> "Menopause is a good time to experiment more with new sexual positions. Positions that give you more control of the depth of penetration and tempo of sex will make it more comfortable for you.
>
> "Spend more time building up to intercourse by hugging, kissing, massaging, and orally stimulating your vagina to give it the extra time it needs to get moist after menopause. Or skip intercourse altogether and spend time discovering new erogenous zones and ways of obtaining mutual pleasure. There is no one right way to be sexual. The intimacy of touch and physical closeness can be as satisfying, if not more so, as intercourse. In fact, for many women it is preferable.
>
> But if intercourse is important to you now or it will be in the future:
>
> "You can prevent some of the changes in your vagina by remaining sexually active after menopause. Vaginal intercourse, masturbation, fantasy, erotic massage, or any other activity that arouses you and gives you sexual pleasure can help to keep your vagina moist, soft, and healthy. Having regular intercourse (once or twice a week or more) or placing a vibrator, dilator, or two or three fingers in your vagina while masturbating once a week will prevent the shortening and shrinking of your vagina that can occur over time when estrogen is lacking. Kegel exercises have also been known to be effective in keeping your vagina toned and elastic."[50]

Much of the time painful intercourse is caused by vaginal dryness, but it also could be caused by tight pelvic floor muscles or even a combination of vaginal dryness and tight muscles. Pain could also be caused by skin conditions, nerve problems, endometriotis, or other reasons, but these are more complicated and less common. An experienced pelvic floor physical therapist can identify muscle problems and can treat and reduce pain. But some of these other conditions need to be treated by a physician.

---

[50] Hilda Hutcherson, *What Your Mother Never Told You About Sex* (New York: Perigee, 2003), 274.

> **Join the Revolution!** Make a "Menopause Plan" in your thirties or early forties!
>
> Just as many women make a "birthing plan" before they go into labor, they should make a "menopause plan" to plan for the different paths they may go down when they hit menopause. And just as women often change their minds when they are in the "heat of the moment" in childbirth, a woman may change her plan depending on what happens during perimenopause. But the bottom line is to think about what you may want to consider when you are going through perimenopause. Some women go through it like a breeze and others suffer. It is better to prepare for the worst and then be pleasantly surprised.
>
> How do you make a plan? First, speak with your doctor. Speak with friends who are in perimenopause and who have already gone through menopause. Make sure to speak with women who have had both good and bad experiences. Ask for advice. Read books on the topic. For example read *The Hormone Decision* by Tara Parker-Pope or see the movie *Hot Flash Havoc*. Or go to the *Hot Flash Havoc* website to read the research by the experts they have collected.[51]
>
> Just as with everything else in life, you may make a plan and then change it when you are going through the reality of the situation. Or you may prepare for the worst and end up asking yourself why you spent all that time when it really wasn't all that bad. But at least you will have prepared and thought about it beforehand instead of being taken by surprise.
>
> ---
> 51 *Hot Flash Havoc: A Film of Menopausal Proportions* website http://www.hotflashhavoc.net/page.cfm?pageid=19156.

CG: Other symptoms and changes happen in menopause as well that we didn't really go over. Many women experience weight gain. Some experience fatigue, hair loss, memory lapses, mood swings, and all kinds of other symptoms. A lot of women get sad or depressed, and sometimes they just feel angry or betrayed by their bodies, or unbalanced. Some women may feel a sense of loss. Many women commiserate with their partners and friends over what is happening. Some seek the help of counselors and others to help them talk through the changes. Some seek the advice of doctors to see if any of the changes are being caused by something else going on in the body like maybe another medical condition. I say, do all of the above. Just like any other time when we go through big changes, menopause is sometimes difficult and sometimes wonderful, and often just very confusing.

And there is also a lot of beauty and grace in it. As Betty Friedan said, "Aging is not lost youth but a new stage for opportunity and strength."

Your Vagina After Cancer

CG: One other topic we need to touch on is the changes that a woman's vagina goes through if a woman has or has had cancer.

LL: Cancer has become so real to me over the past five years. Three of my dear friends have all fought cancer—ovarian, breast, and stomach cancer—and I have seen them fight bravely. My friends have impressed me tremendously. They took what they learned and started research foundations (my closest friend from college, Debbie Zelman, started Can't Stomach Cancer), wrote books (like *But I Just Grew Out My Bangs!: A Cancer Tale*), and volunteered as Chemo Buddies. So after all of that how could I possibly approach them to ask them to tell me what happened with their vaginas while they were going through their cancer ordeals and chemotherapy?

CG: Did you?

LL: Of course I did! But luckily these are my friends who are very open and not so private. My friend Katya, especially—her book has pictures of her breasts right after her original ones were removed, and her new breasts were reconstructed. And she is so open and so funny throughout the book. At one point she talked about how she was having a conversation with her OB/GYN, who is also a friend of hers. She had just gone through surgery where she had her ovaries and uterus removed and said to him that (after she thanked him for discovering her cancer) "Well, I'll at least be much better about seeing you from now on." He answered "You don't need to see me *at all* anymore—you have *nothing for me!*" In the course of three months she had had her ovaries, uterus, and both breasts removed—it didn't occur to her that she had no more use for an OB/GYN.

CG: I can see that—women are so conditioned to see their OB/GYNs or family doctors or internists once a year so they can get a pap smear and a check-up. By the way, there are new guidelines now about how often you need to get a pap test.

Here are the new guidelines from the National Cancer Institute at the National Institutes of Health[52]:

> **Pap and Human Papillomavirus (HPV) Testing Guidelines**
> - Cervical cancer screening, which includes the Pap test and HPV testing, is an essential part of a woman's routine health care because it can detect cancer or abnormalities that may lead to cancer of the cervix.
> - Current guidelines recommend that women should have a Pap test every three years beginning at age twenty-one. These guidelines further recommend that women ages thirty to sixty-five should have HPV and Pap cotesting every five years or a Pap test alone every three years. Women with certain risk factors may need to have more frequent screening or to continue screening beyond age sixty-five. Ask your doctor if you have one of these risk factors.
> - Women who have received the HPV vaccine still need regular cervical screening.

But even though many women no longer need pap tests every year, it is very important for them to still see their doctor once a year for a wellness visit.

I came across a blog recently called MiddlesexMD and the author Dr. Barb DePree published a beautiful blog on this topic. She gave us permission to reprint the blog:

---

52 National Cancer Institute at the National Institutes of Health, accessed November 2012, http://www.cancer.gov/cancertopics/factsheet/detection/Pap-HPV-testing.

After Cancer: Take Care of Your Vagina[53]

November 4, 2011 by Dr. Barb Depree

Whether you were already menopausal or were abruptly deposited into menopause after treatment for your cancer, you're probably familiar with what happens to your vagina when you lose estrogen.

You may experience the burning, itching pain of thin, dry vaginal walls and fragile skin on your genitals. You don't lubricate like you used to, so sex can be difficult or painful. Or, if you're experiencing the muscle spasms of vaginismus, sex may be impossible. Less estrogen is a good thing for some cancer treatments, but it's darned tough on the vagina and, by extension, on your sex life as well.

So, while vaginal health is important for all women during menopause, it's critical for those undergoing cancer treatment. Your vagina and pelvic floor need a lot of TLC right now to stay comfortable and responsive. Fortunately, compared to the other things going on in your life, taking care of your bottom is usually straightforward and inexpensive. Besides, keeping your vagina in good shape might eliminate one problem area and allow you to stay in touch with your sexual self, too.

Consider this four-part approach to caring for your vagina and pelvic floor.

First, use vaginal moisturizers and lubricants.

Moisturizers are your first line of defense. These are nonhormonal, over-the-counter products that are intended to keep your vagina hydrated and to restore a more natural pH balance. They should be used two or three times a week, just as you'd moisturize any other part of your body. Replens, Yes, and Emerita are examples of moisturizers.

Using moisturizers is important whether or not you're having intercourse. It should just be part of a regular health maintenance regimen.

---

[53] Barb Depree, "After Cancer: Take Care of Your Vagina," MiddlesexMDBlog, accessed November 2012, http://blog.middlesexmd.com/2011/11/04/after-cancer-take-care-of-your-vagina/.

Use lubricants liberally before intercourse, on sex toys such as vibrators, and any time you touch the delicate tissue on your genitalia. Also apply lubricant to your partner's penis.

At this point, keep your lubricants plain and simple—no scents or flavors; avoid warming lubes. Don't use any product with glycerin, which can create an environment conducive to yeast infections, and don't use petroleum-based lubricants.

Second, keep your pelvic floor toned. "The pelvic floor is really important in keeping your internal organs in place, preventing incontinence, and enhancing sexual pleasure," says Maureen Ryan, nurse practitioner and sex therapist.

Plus, knowing how to relax your pelvic floor muscles is helpful if you're experiencing the involuntarily spasms of vaginismus.

Kegel exercises, in which you flex and relax the muscles around your vagina, will tone the pelvic floor. Or, you can purchase exercise tools to tone your pelvic floor muscles. This is a great way to make sure you're exercising the right muscles.

Third, use dilators if your vaginal capacity is compromised. Dilators are cylinders that come in sets with various sizes. They're meant to gradually increase the size and capacity of the vaginal opening, which can be important, especially after some cancer surgeries and treatments that constrict the vaginal opening or create scars and adhesions.

To some extent, dilators are helpful just to reassure you that you can tolerate something in your vagina again.

Start with the smallest size dilator, lubricate it, and gently insert it as far in as you can tolerate. Try doing kegel exercises, tensing and relaxing your pelvic floor muscles. Can you feel your muscles close around the dilator? Keep it in for maybe ten minutes and repeat this exercise several times a week. Move on to the next largest size when you can tolerate it.

Fourth, use a vibrator (lubricated, of course). Self-stimulation increases blood flow to your genitals and helps reacquaint you with the feelings and sensations of your body. The more stimulation you can bring to the area, the healthier it will be.

> The point is to keep the vulvo-vaginal area moist and flexible, to increase blood flow, to stay responsive, to maintain capacity, so that when you and your honey are ready to start your engines, you'll both enjoy a smooth ride.

Suggested Resources:

Hot Flash Havoc: A Film of Menopausal Proportions website http://www.hotflashhavoc.net/page.cfm?pageid=19156.

Love, Susan, *Dr. Susan Love's Menopause and Hormone Book: Making Informed Choices* (New York: Three Rivers Press, 2003).

MiddlesexMD Blog: Sexuality for Life-Info, advice and products for women over 40. Excellent blog by Dr. Barb Depree. http://blog.middlesexmd.com/

Norsigian, Judy and Boston Women's Health Book Collective, *Our Bodies, Ourselves: Menopause* (New York: Touchstone, 2006).

Northrup, Christiane, *The Wisdom of Menopause: Creating Physical and Emotional Health During the Change*, revised ed. (New York: Bantam, 2012).

Parker-Pope, Tara, *The Hormone Decision* (New York: Pocket Books, 2008).

Norsigian, Judy and Boston Women's Health Book Collective, *Our Bodies, Ourselves: Menopause* (New York: Touchstone, 2006).

> I would like to make one recommendation for every woman who is approaching menopause. The Boston Women's Health Initiative, the women who wrote *Our Bodies, Ourselves*, also wrote this book on menopause, and I cannot share even one iota of information in just a few pages compared to how much they packed into this book. It is truly fabulous. Here is the link: http://www.ourbodiesourselves.org/publications/menopause/toc.asp.

PART II

VAGINA—THE MIND

12. Sexuality and Physical Intimacy
13. Masturbation
14. Fantasy and Your Biggest Sex Organ — Your Brain!
15. Orgasm
16. Sex

PART II

VAGINA—THE MIND

"[F]or there is nothing either good or bad, but thinking makes it so."

—Shakespeare, *Hamlet* (2.2.11), based on Epictetus

LL: A quick conversation with readers

Before I begin this section, I want to tell you what I am thinking about when I say "Vagina—The Mind." I mean, the vagina is obviously a separate organ from the mind. Since this idea is more abstract, I wanted to tell you where I am going with it and give you a roadmap for this section of the book.

So what does the vagina have to do with the mind? The way we feel about our vaginas, our bodies, our sexuality, and more started at birth—or really before our birth because our parents and communities had many values and ideas about the human body and sexuality before we even came into the world. When we were born, we started soaking up ideas, values, and even energy (either positive or negative or both) from our parents, communities, culture, and more.

Some women grow up thinking very positively about their vaginas. Others are not so lucky. I have one older friend named Gloria (not her real name) who grew up with a mother who smelled her fingers every night before she went to bed and every morning when she woke up. Her mother said that touching her vagina (she didn't actually use that word, just motioned to that part of her anatomy) was evil, and she should stay away from it. Not surprisingly, Gloria grew up with a negative view of her vagina—it was "evil," "dirty," "bad." And it took her years of unlearning this negativity, as well as two failed marriages, before she was able to start thinking of her vagina and her body, as well as her sexuality, positively.

Most examples of this are not so cut and dried. Many women grow up with their mothers never talking about vaginas, or if they do, what is said is not very positive (though it also may not be negative). Even women whose parents don't purposefully send negative messages may do so without meaning it. If a body part like the vagina is not named or if it is given a nickname, then girls may interpret this to mean that it is not proper to talk about their vaginas or think about them or look at them. How many readers have not looked at their own vaginas? I know many women who have not looked at their vaginas for years—if ever. You may ask why this is so bad, and *in and of itself* it may not be, but many of these thoughts lead to other behaviors that can do harm such as not feeling comfortable talking to your doctor about issues involving your vagina, or not being fulfilled in a relationship because you are unable to let go and feel sexual. Many of these learned behaviors, including giving a vagina another name or not looking at your vagina, are very connected to your subconscious thoughts and feelings about your vagina.

One of my favorite quotes relates to this idea. "The last thing a fish would ever notice would be water,"[54] meaning that culture is so pervasive that we just take it for granted. We are often unaware of the context in which we live. We don't

---

54 Anthropologist Ralph Linton wisely said this; quoted in Johnnetta B. Cole, *Anthropology for the Nineties* (New York: Simon & Schuster, 1988), 4.

really think about the "rules" or norms of our own environment or culture unless something changes to make us aware or "get us thinking."

An example of this is for much of the twentieth century in the United States it was a "rule" that African Americans sat in the back of the bus and not in the front, they could not use the same water fountains as white Americans, and so on. When we read about this today many of us cringe thinking how terrible and unfair. But in the 1920s, '30s, '40s, '50s, and so on most white Americans did not cringe thinking about this or even enforcing these rules. They just accepted it and did not question this lifestyle. Thankfully, today, the norm has changed. But if a child was born in the 1940s and saw that this was how life was, and it was just one of the many rules, then he or she usually did not question this. It was just how life went. It was how people were. It was the culture, the "norm."

There were many, many people who did see this as being unfair. They were highly offended by this injustice, and many people fought to do something about it. But they were in the minority; the majority of Americans in the 1950s still wanted to keep schools segregated (with most of the resources going to white schools and the hand-me-downs going to black schools), keep buses segregated, and generally keep the status quo. They weren't necessarily "bad" people who were "hateful" (though some were). They were just brought up this way, and they were taught that this was "normal." Everyone they knew and loved—their parents, friends, and teachers—went along with the status quo, so they did not question it. Just like the last thing a fish would notice would be water, the last thing many humans notice and think about is our own surroundings and the culture we live in and the "norms" we grow up with and believe.

It was not until the tides of social change turned that a majority of people realized how wrong the culture was. This is also fairly "normal." If someone is living in a culture where things like discrimination are a given and then more and more people start understanding that this discrimination is wrong, it is easier for people to catch on to the new way of thinking. It is easier for them to start to question things themselves. I can imagine a white woman in her thirties back in the '50s living in, say, New Jersey. She grows up being taught that blacks are a certain way, and she grows up going to separate schools. She doesn't ever really interact with any black students or have any black friends, so she believes what her parents and teachers tell her. Then she starts hearing some positive messages about black people. Her friends start questioning their own opinions and values and ideas, and she does as well. After all, she is not a closed-minded, hardheaded person. She is just relying on what she has been taught for thirty or more years. But she starts to look at the black woman in the grocery store in a new way. She starts to feel badly that this woman's children are going to a school where they have textbooks that are falling apart (or no textbooks at all) when she knows her own children are at a brand-new school with brand-new textbooks. She even starts to wonder what her children would be like if they grew up in a black family, and she wonders what it would be like if the sweet little black boy in the park were actually her child. She starts questioning her values and questioning her way of thinking. She starts to *think about* the water she is surrounded by—or rather the air, the culture, the norms, the values. And she starts to decide that they are *not fair*.

This might seem like an extreme example, but we still live in a society and culture and environment whose rules we do not question. This is just human. How could we live if we were always questioning everything? For example, if you had to think about everything you did all day long…should we really be eating meat when the poor animals are defenseless[55]? Should we really be putting people to death using the death penalty when data have shown that it is unjust? Is it fair to own a dog when we don't have enough time to walk or play with our dog? Are we using the best parenting techniques with our children[56]? Am I eating foods or doing other things that can cause cancer like using my cell phone? If we had to constantly question everything, we would never be able to live our lives. So humans purposely block out many messages they get and many thoughts they have in order to have room in their brains for daily living.

The last thing a fish thinks about is water. The last thing we think about is the givens of the society we were brought up in—that is unless we learn to question things and become independent thinkers. We don't always have time and energy to do this…but for some really important things, if we did take the time to question, to dig, to grow and develop in certain areas, it would make a major, profound difference in our lives and the lives of our families, friends and loved ones.

CG: OK, I just have to interrupt you for one minute. (I know you are talking to the readers, but I am listening, too.) Where are we going with this? What does this have to do with vaginas?

LL: Ha! Sorry, I had to set that up because this is a really important topic, and it needs some pre-explanation. What do our vaginas have to do with our minds? Just about everything.

---

55 I eat meat. I just know that many people feel this way, and they do have a point.
56 My father always says, "I used to have six parenting theories and no children…now I have six children and no theories!"

VAGINA—THE MIND

The way we feel about our vaginas, our bodies and our sexuality started at birth, when we began soaking up ideas, values, and even energy from our parents, communities and the world.

WHAT I MEAN BY THE *MIND*

When I am talking about our *minds* I am talking about our brains, our thoughts, and our ideas. There are lots of scientists, psychologists, and philosophers who argue over what our minds are. For example, is the mind just our brain, the physical part of our body that is inside our skull? Or is the mind the *only* thing that actually exists, and is the external world just an illusion created by the mind?

This can get way too philosophical. There are whole books, *volumes* written on what people mean when they say "the mind." In this book, when I talk about the *mind*, I am talking about **how you use your brain to process information, both consciously and subconsciously**. There are lots of subconscious thoughts, ideas, and feelings lurking in our brains, and they greatly influence our conscious thoughts, ideas, and values. But the *mind* also includes the conscious part—where you think and make decisions, where you can think about your ideas and values and even decide to consciously change them if you put your mind to it...

Here's one example of how you <u>consciously</u> use your brain. I have my period and need some tampons and pads. I go to Target and look though the aisle...hmmm...*I always get the same pads because I know what works well for a lighter flow and for a heavy, nighttime flow. But those tampons – the last ones I tried were a bit painful going in. Hmm, I'll try a different brand this time.* So I buy the same pads and a different kind of tampon.

Here's an example of how your <u>subconscious</u> affects your brain. *She has her period, and she is on the last few pads and tampons. She knows she needs to buy more, but she feels so ambivalent. She really hates using tampons. But she doesn't know one single person who only uses pads, and they are so much messier. But she hates putting tampons in – always has. She tries different brands, but she always finds something wrong with them. The last ones really hurt when they went in.* And then <u>consciously</u> she decides, *All right, I'll buy these new ones...but maybe I should just use the pads. Maybe I should run back to the pad section and get a few more kinds of pads for medium, daytime flow.*

> Since I have a counseling background, I cannot possibly think of the subconscious and conscious minds as separate. Rather, I see them working together very closely. For example, a child whose parents recently got divorced may start acting up more in class, but she may not realize she is acting up because of her internal pain and anguish. She may blame herself, have lower self-esteem as a result, and then start telling herself that she is bad, and she doesn't deserve to have good friends or a boyfriend or good grades. Her subconscious influences her conscious, and her thoughts turn this into a self-fulfilling prophecy. She acts out, talks back to her teachers, and is mean to her friends.
>
> As humans, we have lots of subconscious thoughts that have been shaped by years of experience, upbringing, culture, and more. When we try to understand these subconscious thoughts, we can better understand why we think the thoughts we think and why we behave the way that we do. The mind plays a huge role in the person we are and can also help us become the person we want to be.

TRY THIS EXERCISE: A GUIDED MEDITATION

One thing I find really helpful for getting started with knowing and exploring our subconscious minds is this guided visualization we use with teenagers in the human sexuality class I help teach. This guided meditation helps us shake up that water and make us realize that maybe we have certain thoughts, emotions, and beliefs surrounding our vaginas because of our upbringing, culture, or community. It is an enlightening way to realize just how many messages we have stuck in our brains that are actually not *our own* messages, but rather ones we *picked up from our environment*. Maybe we have never taken the time to think for ourselves and come to our own conclusions about some of these topics.

Before reading this, get comfortable and cozy. Maybe dim the lights, light a candle. Even consider having a loved one read it out loud to you so you can close your eyes and listen and think. Read it slowly and with feeling. This may take about ten minutes to read.

Copyright Pamela Wilson and Wayne Pawlowski, Sexuality Trainers, Metropolitan Washington, DC, 1999

Modified by Elizabeth Casparian and Eva Goldfarb, 1999 ed., Cantor Andrew Bernard, 2009

Guided Meditation

Think back…as far as you can remember…to when you were a young child. Try to picture the home that you grew up in, especially your bedroom or wherever you slept.

Picture your parents or guardians…how did they feel about your birth, and how did you know? Were they happy about you being a biological boy or girl? How did you know?

Now picture the other people who may have lived with you…sisters or brothers and any other relatives or close friends. Picture their faces. How did all of those family members get along? How much communication was there in your family? How much affection was shown, and how was it shown?

Do you remember your family getting together with other relatives?

How did your family celebrate birthdays? What rituals or traditions do you remember most?

Are there any special toys you played with, or was there any special object that you were particularly attached to when you were a young child?

Do you remember your first experience with school? What do you remember about kindergarten? Do you remember the classroom, the teacher, the playground, or anything else important?

Try to remember the first time you realized that the world was divided into males and females, and what that meant to you. Try to remember the first time you realized you were biologically male or female and how this felt.

Did you like being a girl? Did you like being a boy? Did you feel like you were born to be the gender you looked like to the outside world?

When you were very young, what names were you taught for the sexual parts of your body such as your vulva, vagina, and breasts, or penis, scrotum, and testicles? What feelings or attitudes did you develop about those parts? For example, were they good or bad…clean or dirty…secret or OK to talk about?

Do you remember touching and exploring your own body when you were young? What is the youngest age you remember doing so? Did anyone ever find you touching yourself? If so, how did they react and how did you feel?

Did you ever play touching games with other kids? If you did, did you play them openly or secretly, and why? In addition, what did these games mean to you…and to the kids you played with?

Were your parents or guardians physically affectionate with each other? How did they express their feelings in your presence? Did they use sexual words in front of you? Did you sense that they were comfortable talking about sex or not? How could you tell?

Where did you first learn about intercourse? Who told you? When did it first occur to you that your parents had intercourse together, and what did you think about this?

When, if ever, did your parents or guardians first speak directly to you about sexuality? What were those conversations like for you and for them?

As you got older, how did you feel about your body changing? How did you feel about your hips and breasts getting larger? Did you worry that your penis was too small or too large? Who did you talk with about these changes and concerns?

If you are disabled, how did this impact how you experienced your sexual development? Your gender identity? How other people treated you with respect to sex and gender?

How did you learn about menstruation…orgasms…or wet dreams? Who told you, and what did they tell you? How did you feel about the information? How did you feel when you had your first period? When you had your first orgasm or wet dream? Did you tell anyone about these events? Why or why not?

If there were boys and girls in your family, were there any differences in the way your parents raised you? Did they give you any different messages about sex and proper sexual behavior? What were these differences, and how did you feel about them?

Try to remember the first time you felt overtly and consciously sexually attracted to someone. Can you remember who it was? Picture that person and try to recreate your feelings. What did you do with your feelings? If the person was someone you knew, how did you behave around him or her? Did you tell anyone about your feelings? Why or why not?

When do you remember being aware that people had boyfriends or girlfriends? When you were growing up, did you date? Whether you did or you didn't, what were the reasons? If you did date, how far sexually would you go on dates, and how did you decide where to draw the line?

Did you masturbate as you got older? If you did, how did you feel physically and emotionally? Who taught you how to masturbate? Do you remember when you had your first orgasm? What was that like? If you've never had an orgasm, what is that like for you?

Try to remember your first noncoercive, erotic sexual contact with another person. Who was it with? Why did you do it? How did you feel physically and emotionally about it?

When did you first hear and understand the words heterosexual… homosexual…bisexual? Transgender? Intersex? When did you first clearly and consciously associate one or more of those words with you? How did you feel when you did? Who did you talk to about this?

What messages did you receive about marriage and commitment? How did those messages affect your future relationships?

Think forward in time to the present. How comfortable are you with sexuality today?

Sweep over all the memories that you have just revisited. What are some of the ways that your race, ethnicity, and culture have influenced your sexuality?

Now slowly return to this space…and open your eyes when you are ready.

LL: I am always overwhelmed by the power of that guided meditation. It is very powerful and quite comprehensive, and it is a great way to realize exactly how much our minds influence our feelings about ourselves, our sexuality, our identity, and our vaginas. And it often brings up so many memories and emotions...even a few tears. This is an effective tool for self-exploration, and I could also imagine couples or friends using it to get to know each other better. Book clubs can even use it as an activity.

It gets to the root of so many of our assumptions and biases. By reading it and thinking about how you grew up and the messages you got, compared to how your friends and family and partner grew up, and the messages they might have been getting, you can see how women have so many different attitudes and thoughts about all of these topics.

The messages some women get lead them to think of their bodies as temples, while others get messages that lead them to think of themselves as dirty. It is why one person feels shameful when thinking about sex while another feels adventurous. All of this is so important to how we feel about ourselves, our bodies, our sexuality, and whether or not we deserve to be happy (we all do, btw).

The bottom line is that if you are entirely happy with how you feel about your vagina, your body, and your sexuality, that is wonderful. You can skip this next section and meet us in the next chapter called Physical Intimacy. But even women who are totally comfortable may have some subconscious shame or some shame they are unaware of. If you are not comfortable with your body, there are ways of reversing old messages you might not have liked and changing your feelings, thoughts, and behaviors—in essence, *changing your mind.*

WHEN YOU CHANGE YOUR MIND, YOU CHANGE YOUR WORLD

We just read that old messages can really affect your current thinking. But the good news is that your mind is very trainable. If you don't like the old messages, or if you don't like your current behaviors or feelings, you can train yourself and literally change your mind, changing the messages you send to yourself.

My close friend Dr. Rebecca Fleischer, who is a clinical psychologist in the D.C. area, has a really fabulous way of diagramming the mind and showing how emotions can affect your thoughts from your mind, which can then translate to behaviors. *Becky's triangle*, as I like to call it, shows how our thoughts, behaviors, and emotions all affect one another and are interrelated. Some women are more comfortable operating more cognitively and some more emotionally, but all three are always affecting each other to some degree. By the way, if you have done any work with a counselor, or if you are familiar with cognitive behavioral therapy, then this will likely look familiar.

This relationship can be diagrammed like a big triangle with arrows pointing in both directions. Each of the three areas affects the other two. They are all interrelated, like this:

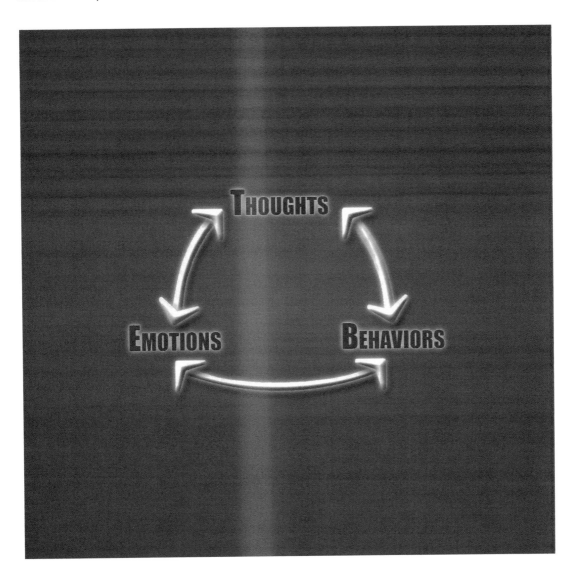

The basic premise of cognitive behavioral therapy (Becky's triangle) is this:

An event happens (let's say Lisa is dating David, and he makes a comment about wanting to change something in their sex lives—let's just say he wants her to initiate sex more).

This triggers an emotion in Lisa's brain. She had previous bad experiences with men who were controlling or who wanted her to change, and those experiences were very hurtful. When David asks her to change something, she experiences negative emotions, and that triggers something else—negative thoughts.

She starts to think to herself, "I am such a loser, sexually speaking...I can't seem to do anything right, and I can't seem to make my partner happy...no wonder I've had so many failed relationships." These negative thoughts start to trigger something else—negative behaviors.

Lisa starts to pull away from David. Instead of initiating sex more, as he asked her to, she starts making excuses for why she doesn't want to have sex. She does not want to experience those painful feelings again, so she does this to protect herself. But it has the opposite effect—it starts to hurt her relationship with David.

Now what is really going on here? From David's perspective, he is in a relationship with a really fabulous woman, he is getting to know her better and better, and he really likes being intimate with her. But in the past, he had a two-year relationship with Margot, and she never initiated sex—it was always up to him. He started to think that Margot really wasn't attracted to him, and that was part of what caused the relationship to end. He decided that when he got into a relationship with another woman, he would be more up-front about this if he needed to be. So when he asked Lisa in a kind way if she could please initiate sex more, he thought he was being proactive and helping the relationship along.

HOW DOES LISA CHANGE HER THOUGHTS?

First, she needs to recognize them. If she starts to feel hurt when David asks her to initiate sex more, she needs to talk to herself and ask herself, "Is it that he doesn't like me sexually, or is it that he wants to get one of his own needs met?" Then she should ask herself, "Is this a reasonable request?" She also needs to recognize when her hurt emotions trigger negative thoughts about herself. Once this is recognized, she needs to replace these negative thoughts with positive ones like "I am a very sexual person, and I like sex...men enjoy having sex with me…my other relationships did not work out because there were other things wrong, and they were just not meant to be…" Replacing negative thoughts with positive ones requires a lot of work, but it is worth it. The hard work includes constant reminders to yourself to do this. When someone changes her thoughts, she can literally change her world. For example, if Lisa took those positive thoughts and (if she wanted to) started to initiate sex more—after all, she really likes David, and she is very happy with the rest of the relationship—then this could only help their relationship blossom even more.

IF EXPLORING EMOTIONS MAKES YOU FEEL UNCOMFORTABLE

Some women (and you know who you are!) don't like delving into the world of emotions and feelings and especially don't like examining their triggers. Others are uberemotional and can read self-help books all day long. Yet more fall in between these two groups. If you are happy with how you are, that is great. Changing your mind and changing your thoughts should only be something you approach if there is something about your life that you want to change. If that is the case, I also suggest working with a counselor or therapist on this—they can be so helpful in helping you identify your triggers and practice changing your thoughts.

LL: OK, now back to the chapters. In Vagina—the Mind we take a look at Physical Intimacy and how it relates to the vagina. Then we move on to Fantasy and Your Biggest Sex Organ—Your Brain. In this chapter we talk about how so many of the messages I wrote about above can affect your feelings about intimacy and sexuality. Then we home in more on masturbation and orgasm, and we conclude with a chapter on sex.

Suggested Resources:

Ensler, Eve, *The Vagina Monologues* (New York: Random House, 2007).

Hite, Shere, *The Hite Report: A National Study of Female Sexuality* (New York: Seven Stories Press, 2003).

Wolf, Naomi, *Vagina: A New Biography* (New York: Ecco, 2012).

CHAPTER 12

Sexuality and Physical Intimacy

LL note to readers: When I started to write about vaginas, I knew that in addition to just the anatomy, there was so much to learn and explore when it came to vaginas and intimacy. And when I say intimacy, I mean all kinds of more-than-friendship feelings and touching with another human being. I asked my good friend Lenore to help me with this chapter because she is a retired sex therapist, she collects erotic art, and she is an all-around brilliant and insightful woman. Also, she did much of her work with couples and intimacy. Lenore is also wrapped into the composite expert CG, as are other health and mental health professionals.

LL: First, why are intimacy and sex important? I think most adults can agree that they are. But why?

CG: You pose a good question—why is all of this important? Why is intimacy important? Why is sexuality important? I think the bottom line is that intimacy is so salient because it fulfills a basic human need, and sex is important because it also fulfills a basic human need. Plus it is a significant component of most committed relationships. And both are healthy, both physiologically and psychologically.

LL: Finally something that feels good is also good for you!

CG: Definitely. Before getting into it here, we should first define the difference between an intimate relationship, physical intimacy, sexuality, and sex itself:

Definition of Physical Intimacy

Intimate relationships make the world go 'round. Human beings have an internal drive to belong and to love, and this is often satisfied within an intimate relationship. "Intimate relationships involve physical and sexual attraction by one person to another, liking and loving, romantic feelings, and sexual relationships, as well as the seeking of a mate and emotional and personal support of each other."[57]

A relationship can be *physically intimate* without being sexual per se. For example, imagine two younger teens who have budding sexual feelings for each other, but they are not yet at a place where they are exploring sexually. They may express physical intimacy by holding hands or putting their arms around each other. Another example is the intimacy between parents and children. This is possible at any age. If two people have a relationship where they express their intimacy physically, with their bodies, then it is considered physical intimacy.

Physical intimacy is also highly correlated with *sexuality*, where two people explore each other's bodies more deeply and satisfy each other's sexual longings. The American Psychological Association (APA) further breaks down *sexuality* into the following three different stages. <u>Desire</u> is

---

[57] Rowland Miller and Daniel Perlman, *Intimate Relationships*, 5th ed., (New York: McGraw-Hill, 2008).

an interest in being sexual, Excitement is the state of arousal that sexual stimulation causes, and Orgasm is sexual pleasure's peaking.[58] The APA goes on to say that a sexual disorder occurs when there is a problem in at least one of these stages. But I think that this sounds harsh and scary. Sometimes it is just a small thought change[59] that can "fix" this "disorder," though other times it requires more.

We define *sex* as either oral sex (when one partner's mouth comes into contact with the other partner's genitals), anal sex (in which a penis goes into the partner's anus), masturbation (touching or rubbing one's own genitals), and vaginal intercourse (penis in vagina if you are heterosexual, or if you are a lesbian, then either *tribbing*[60] or fingers or anything else in each other's vagina). But when I talk about sex, I always try to be as specific as possible—for example, if I mean intercourse, I will say intercourse, and if I mean oral sex, I will say oral sex.

---

58 "Sexuality," *American Psychological Association*, 2012, accessed October 2012, http://www.apa.org/topics/sexuality/index.aspx.
59 Refer back to Becky's triangle.
60 Tribadism (or tribbing) is a form of nonpenetrative sex in which a woman rubs her vulva against her partner's body for sexual stimulation. More information on lesbian sex is in the chapter on sex.

Evolution of Physical Intimacy and Sexuality

CG: Sexual exploration starts at birth. Babies touch their genitals because it feels good. Sexual exploration is part of how we see ourselves, what messages we get about our bodies, how we want others to see us, what we learn about being male or female, what we feel sexually throughout our lives, the decisions we make in relationships about our sexual behavior, and more.

In a perfect world, a girl grows up appreciating and exploring her own body. She likes how it feels when she touches her genitals. She goes through a period of discovery when she is younger. Some girls press down on their vulvas, almost like a precursor to masturbation. When a girl presses down, she can feel pressure against her clitoris and the clitoral shaft, and it feels good. Girls and babies can even bring themselves to orgasm.

As she gets older, she may experiment with others, either boys or girls, depending on her sexual orientation or inclination at that moment. It usually starts with older children or younger teenagers developing crushes on each other and flirting with each other. It then typically escalates to holding hands. A woman's skin (a man's, too) is the largest organ of the body, and it carries a network of very sensitive nerve endings all over the body. So sometimes we become aroused just by holding hands or touching a shoulder or a cheek. Really, any part of your body could be stimulated for sexual arousal.

Sometimes we express intimacy by holding hands or touching someone's arm or looking into their eyes. Intimacy is not only physical but it is also emotional. We may share a secret with someone we feel intimate with, and this act shows the other person how much we care about and trust them, or vice versa.

A girl or woman may kiss someone and feel butterflies in her stomach or a warm feeling in her genitals or in the genital area, and that is the beginning of sexual desire. Any parts of our body that are sensitive to sensual touch—not just the sexual parts of our anatomy—are called erogenous zones. For both women and men, this may include the back of the neck, the inner ear, fingers, feet, inner thighs, mouths, and tongues, and of course the more obvious parts like nipples and genitalia.

When a young woman is involved with someone, she may experiment with kissing and touching her partner's erogenous zones and see how different parts of her body feel in response to touch. At the same time, she may take in the reaction of her partner when she touches his or her erogenous zones. She may go further—maybe her partner will feel her breasts, and she may touch her partner's penis or vagina. They may explore other areas as well like oral sex. She may enjoy receiving oral sex, where her partner licks and sucks on her vulva. She may enjoy giving oral sex. Or she may not enjoy oral sex. The important part of sexual exploration is exploring with a partner who makes her feel safe and comfortable. Often, when women (and men) explore sexually, they feel very vulnerable. If a woman's partner says something mean about a body part or performance when she is feeling vulnerable, it can really stick. It is not always true that sticks and stones will break your bones, but words will never hurt you—as can be attested by many women who have been hurt by their partners' words. It is not the body parts that remain in pain, it is the mind. Often we replay the mean words over in our minds, and they affect how we feel about our bodies and sexuality.

When a woman is young and exploring, or when she is with a new partner, she learns a great deal about what she likes and what she wants. Yes, she wants her breasts touched and a tongue in her ear but, no, she does not like her butt squeezed, for example.

Unfortunately, she does not always have a chance to explore and find out what feels good and right before she is influenced by the media. Much of what she wants or considers "normal" is formed by what she sees in movies or on TV or reads in books and magazines. Learning to like one sexual act or another is not necessarily congenital or instinctual. This is just like eating. All humans must eat to survive, but if you grow up in the United States or Canada you develop very different food tastes than you do if you grow up in Japan…or India…or Kenya.

LL: That makes me think about what happens when we take our children to a Chinese restaurant and they think that the desserts aren't "real" desserts because they are not chocolate or cake or ice cream. For example, have you ever seen the Chinese dessert called gao? It is a rice-based dessert and often comes in a jelly-like consistency or firm and chewy. Anyway, it does not look at all appealing to my kids. But I am sure kids in China would look at our selection of desserts and ask where the gao is.

CG: That rings very true. In some countries, desserts are just lightly sweetened, whereas in North America they have much more sugar. So we are used to sweeter desserts. Well, similarly, a teenager who has never been involved in a sexual relationship sees a movie with a dramatic, passionate kiss scene, like Kelly McGinnis and Harrison Ford in *Witness,* or a more fun and creative kiss like the upside-down kiss of Kirsten Dunst and Tobey Maguire in *Spider-Man.* And the next thing you know, that is how the teenager imagines kissing someone. If it matches what she has seen on TV or in the movies, it feels "right," and if it doesn't, then perhaps it does not feel right.

With food, what we think is tasty and what we think is gross is culturally determined and learned. So are the things we decide during sexual exploration. This is important to note because it can delay or impede a woman's really getting to know what she likes and what she doesn't like.

And one more thing I just need to say here — the ease of simultaneous orgasm in these Hollywood movies is damaging and inaccurate to say the least! I remember watching *From Here to Eternity* with Burt Lancaster and Deborah Kerr. I think they hurt generations of women who then thought that simultaneous orgasm was the gold standard in sex. More recently in *No Strings Attached,* with Ashton Kutcher and Natalie Portman, they just hop into bed and have a simultaneous orgasm. I did love the fact that they used a condom — that is so important for movie watchers and the public to see because it reinforces what should be happening. But the reality of simultaneous orgasm is that it is very difficult to achieve and does not necessarily mean it is better than another way of being sexually intimate. Some people enjoy having separate orgasms or for others it is not important to have an orgasm. Some people really like being intimate and don't even need to have penetration. To each her own. But I had to add this here because Hollywood and TV images stick in our brain so much and influence how we think our sex lives *should be* and it is just not real.

LL: But Hollywood can also and has also influenced women in a positive way. For example Hollywood has changed our views about masturbation, and Hollywood movies have helped and can continue to help make the topic less taboo and more commonplace. Imagine a really popular movie for say, college-age kids where there is a great masturbation scene by a leading actress. You are saying that something like that can really change the ideas of sexual exploration for a whole generation of women.

CG: Exactly. There have been great masturbation scenes in movies — like Shirley MacLaine in *Being There* in 1979 or Eva Mendes in *We Own the Night* in 2007. But I don't think there has been anything so big and profoundly thought changing…yet.

But back to what I was saying! At a certain point, a teenager or young woman will feel ready to have sexual intercourse.[61] In a perfect world, she would have heard by then that she should use condoms or dental dams[62] to protect against pregnancy and sexually transmitted infections.

> In more recent years the term sexually transmitted infections (STIs) has taken the place of sexually transmitted diseases (STDs) or venereal disease (VD). The new, accepted term is STIs.

Sexual exploration also involves learning to be intimate with someone, not only physically but emotionally. Most girls practice learning about intimacy

---

[61] Forty-nine percent of women have sex by age seventeen and 92 percent by age twenty-four. See W.D. Mosher, A. Chandra and J. Jones, "Sexual Behavior and Selected Health Measures: Men and Women 15–44 Years of Age, United States, 2002," *Advance Data from Vital and Health Statistics*, no. 362 (Hyattsville, MD: National Center for Health Statistics, 2005).

[62] Dental dams can be used during oral sex. A dental dam, like a condom, is a barrier method. It is a thin, square piece of rubber that is placed over the labia or anus during oral-vaginal or oral-anal intercourse. Dental dams are most often made of thin latex rubber; however, they are also available in silicone. Dental dams can be bought in stores like condoms, or they can be made out of plastic wrap or similar materials. A dental dam can help reduce the risk of STI transmission, including herpes, genital warts (HPV), and HIV.

through their childhood, when they share secrets with friends and learn whom to trust and whom not to trust. They also learn to be trustworthy friends and partners if that is something they value.

Hopefully, when they are exploring sexually, they are also continuing to be good friends with their partner and keeping their partner's secrets safe.

So intimacy and sexuality are interrelated and very important background to the next few chapters. Though they may not be highly correlated. For example, many women have one-night stands or casual sex, so they may be physically intimate even when there is no long-term relationship there.

LL: You mentioned earlier that there were many health benefits of being physically intimate and sexually active. I would love to hear about that.

CG: Here are just some of the health benefits. What else can you do (besides maybe exercise and eat well) that can give you all of these physiological *and* psychological health benefits?

Engaging in acts of sexual expression is not only good but good for you!

There is abundant scientific research about the numerous health benefits of being sexual. The list below is taken from *What's Up Down There*, by Dr. Lissa Rankin. Beverly Whipple, PhD., R.N., famed sex researcher and professor emerita from Rutgers University, lists the following evidence-based benefits of sexual expression.[63] Engaging in acts of sexual expression may:

- Help you live longer
- Lower your risk of heart disease and stroke if you have sex at least twice a week
- Reduce your risk of breast cancer
- Bolster your immune system
- Help you sleep
- Make you appear more youthful
- Improve your fitness
- Help protect against endometriosis
- Enhance fertility
- Regulate menstrual cycles

---
63 Rankin, *What's Up Down There? Questions You'd Only Ask Your Gynecologist If She Was Your Best Friend*, 116–117.

- Relieve menstrual cramps
- Help carry a pregnancy to full term
- Relieve chronic pain
- Help reduce migraine headache pain in some individuals
- Improve quality of life
- Reduce the risk of depression
- Lower stress levels
- Improve self esteem
- Improve intimacy with your partner
- Help you grow spiritually

CG: I would venture to say that even if a woman doesn't like sex or want sex, she should still have sex for the health benefits if at all possible. But there is a caveat here. If a woman is not interested in sex, then she should figure out why she is not interested so that she can work on that first.

Reasons why women may not want to have sex

CG: There are so many reasons why women may not be having sex or may not want to have sex. I am going to give you a quick summary and also my medical opinions.

1. **Lack of a partner.** It is healthier for your vagina if you masturbate and have orgasms.

2. **Not liking their partners.** This is really beyond the scope of our book, but if a woman is in an unhealthy relationship, she should look into this. Perhaps start by finding a therapist she can speak with.

3. **Painful intercourse.** This could be caused by many things, including dryness, muscle spasms, or medical conditions like endometriosis or postmenopausal reduction in hormones. I recommend seeing a health care professional who also understands sexuality. Premenopausal intercourse should always be pain free. After menopause there may be additional factors to address like dryness and changes in arousal patterns. Much of this will depend on the quality of the vaginal tissue, how well you lubricate, and how easy it is to get aroused.

4. **Feeling self-conscious about yourself or your body.** There are many things you can do to help yourself feel less self-conscious. First, knowledge is power. Read this and other books to better understand your

body and why it reacts the way it does. Also, intimacy is about trust and relationships, not about appearance. I advise talking to a counselor about this so you are able to feel less self-conscious and able to enjoy intimacy more.

5. **Sexual inhibition.** Did you notice that of the five reasons listed here two of them are more *psychological* (i.e., involve the mind-vagina connection) while one is medical? Our minds play such a big role in whether or not we want to have sex. If a woman is inhibited and does not want to be, she should read books on the topic and talk to a counselor.

LL: I have heard that sex is one of those use-it or lose-it type of things, especially after a woman goes through menopause. Is that true?

CG: I personally do not agree with this, but different experts have different opinions about this. I have a good friend who is an OB/GYN, and she often talks about how the rugae, or the pleats, on the inside of your vagina change over time. She explains that before menopause, the pleats unfold and fold up again easily when a woman engages in sex. The organ is nice and stretchy, thanks to estrogen. After menopause, the natural lubrication may decrease and your nice, stretchy organ gets less flexible as the tissue thins. If your vagina is not "exercised" and regularly stretched out by a penis or vibrator or fingers (helped by lubrication), then it gets less capable and intercourse can be uncomfortable and even more painful if sex is attempted. In the medical world this is called vaginal atrophy.

She also explains that the number one risk factor for painful intercourse is if a woman has not had a baby vaginally. Number two is if she has already gone through menopause, especially if she did not use hormones.

She goes on to say that if a woman's husband or partner has any kind of erectile function problems, this makes intercourse even more difficult, though I have often heard from patients that one benefit of a smaller, softer penis is that it can hurt less.

LL: If a woman is experiencing difficulty or painful intercourse, can she go to her OB/GYN for help?

CG: Her OB/GYN can help in many cases. But just because someone is an OB/GYN does not mean that she is necessarily an expert in sexual functioning. In fact, I would argue that there are not many professionals out there who are good at helping people with sexual functioning. Even marriage and family counselors often need to refer patients to physical therapists or sex therapists, who can often help with painful intercourse.

Sometimes it takes a lot of research because your primary doctor may not even be knowledgeable about who is out in the community doing this kind of work. If a woman is unhappy or experiencing painful sex, she needs to really do research to find the right kind of help.

LL: I think most women who go to see a health care professional about a problem they are experiencing with their vagina would just assume that *any* health care professional would be able to understand and address the issue at hand. However the more I learn about vaginas, the more I realize this is not true.

CG: Yes, just like we discussed in chapter 10, each professional understands a certain aspect of it. Some overlap more than others. For example a good sex therapist will understand the medical problems. A good gynecologist will understand the dermatological diseases. But if a patient presents with a problem, and the problem is not solved by the health care professional she sees, then she should seek out one of the other experts. Here is the Venn diagram from chapter 10 to use as a visual reminder of this. If a problem persists and is not resolved with the help of one professional then seek out the help of a different specialist. Women should not just accept pain or discomfort as something that is a given.

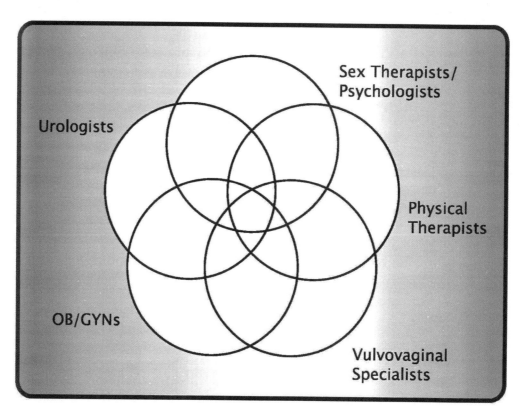

Sometimes the sooner you get help, the better, because if the rugae in your vagina get less stretchy, it may take longer to return to normal function. Every woman is different—there are some women who don't have much of a problem returning to normal function, and others who never quite return.

Some women are comfortable with asking for help in this area, and that is great. But even if a woman is uncomfortable, it is important that she get help for the purposes of her overall health. And again, sooner is better than later.

LL: This is where the whole brain-vagina connection comes in. We've learned that sex is healthy for you and improves your overall health. But if a woman is avoiding sex because she is having trouble or pain and is too shy to say something or to get help, then she could be harming her overall health. If she can become more comfortable with her vagina, her body, and her sexuality, then she can help her overall health. By reading this and other books, going online, and talking to doctors or trusted friends, she can free the energy that might be holding her back and making her feel uncomfortable or ashamed.

CG: Yes, and even if a woman does not have a partner, she can still experience some of these health benefits from having sex by herself.

Suggested Resources:

Barbach, Lonnie, *For Each Other: Sharing Sexual Intimacy* (New York: Anchor, 1983).

Hendrix, Harville, *Getting the Love You Want: A Guide For Couples* (New York: Henry Holt, 2007).

Janus, Samuel S. and Cynthia L. Janus, *The Janus Report on Sexual Behavior* (Hoboken, NJ: John Wiley & Sons, 1993).

Miller, Rowland and Daniel Perlman, *Intimate Relationships* (New York: McGraw-Hill, 2011).

CHAPTER 13

Masturbation

LL: The good news is that just as vaginas are getting more and more press coverage and mentions in movies and television in mainstream culture, so is masturbation.

CG: I'm glad that you say so, but I haven't heard much about it.

LL: Well, the bad news is that there is still a significant amount of shame and embarrassment attached to the term. Sexual norms and taboos don't change overnight. I just read that the National Survey of Sexual Health and Behavior (NSSHB) reported that fifty-eight percent of women don't masturbate regularly.

And the survey and the Kinsey Institute found that of those women who do masturbate, *almost fifty percent feel guilty*.[64]

CG: I'm glad that it is getting more attention because most of the health benefits of having sex apply to masturbation, too. Masturbation helps bolster the immune system, helps relieve stress and pain, and helps you sleep better. So if you don't have a sexual partner, or even if you do, there are actually good health reasons for exploring your own body.

LL: I love hearing that. Something else that feels good is also good *for* you. Finally. Well, masturbation, sex, and dark chocolate. But everything in moderation, I know.

CG: So let's dive right in. Ba-dum-dum.

LL: Speaking of jokes…one of my favorite jokes of all time is the one about the survey about masturbation. It goes something like this.

> So there was a survey of a hundred women, and they were asked if they masturbated…thirty percent said yes.
> And what about the other seventy percent?
> They lied.

Out of curiosity, I looked up the latest research on this topic and found that more than half of women aged eighteen to forty-nine reported masturbating during the previous ninety days. Rates were highest among those from twenty-five to twenty-nine and progressively lower in older age groups.[65] Here is the data broken down by age. This includes the percentages of women who have ever masturbated and also who have masturbated in the past month:

---

[64] Center for Sexual Health Promotion Indiana University, "Special Issue: Findings from the National Survey of Sexual Health and Behavior (NSSHB)," *Journal of Sexual Medicine*, 7, s5 (2010): 243-373.

Weiten, Wayne, Dana S. Dunn and Elizabeth Yost Hammer, *Psychology Applied to Modern Life: Adjustment in the 21st Century*, (Belmont, CA: Wadsworth, 2011), 388.

[65] "Special Issue: Findings from the National Survey of Sexual Health and Behavior," *Journal of Sexual Medicine*, 7, supp. 5 (2010) : 243-373.

AGE of WOMEN[66]	EVER MASTURBATED	PAST MONTH
25–29	85%	52%
30–39	80%	39%
40–49	78%	39%
50–59	77%	28%
60–69	72%	22%
70+	58%	12%

It's important to note that there have been many different, highly respected studies that have asked about masturbation rates in many different ways over the years. When I was doing research for this book I found research results from recent and very reliable sources, but they still show widely different results. That is because they ask different questions in different ways and respondents in some studies are more honest than others, depending on how comfortable they are.

CG: Looking at the data it appears that my generation, women in their fifties, is definitely behind yours, women in their forties, in terms of percentages of women who have masturbated in the past month. But as the data skews younger it shows that more women are masturbating and more frequently as well. For example fifty-two percent of women ages twenty-five to twenty-nine report masturbating in the past month and eighty-five percent of women in that age range reported ever masturbating. Even though as a health care professional I would like to see data that shows that all women masturbate regularly, I am encouraged that in general more and more women are masturbating. Or at least they are admitting it more. They are gaining the health benefits and the stress-busting benefits. And they are also becoming more knowledgeable about how their bodies respond and they can then communicate that to their partners. What is not to like about all of this?

LL: I love it! But I have a deeper question that I have been curious about. Why all the stigma attached to masturbation when it is just a normal, natural thing? Why is there so much shame and guilt attached to it? Why do some people hear the word *masturbation* and just cringe? Why do people sometimes lie to researchers? Why, why, why?

CG: Well, for one thing, there are many subtle messages about vaginas being dirty. There are a lot of parents out there who brought up their children to

---

66   Chart is from the Kinsey Institute at the University of Indiana.

think that touching themselves was shameful. I have had patients tell me that their parents used words with them like "committing the sin of masturbating." Another client was caught masturbating when she was a child and was severely punished. There are some very deeply felt beliefs out there about masturbation.

And then there are all the MYTHS like masturbation stretches out your labia, masturbation makes you unable to have an orgasm vaginally, and even some older myths like masturbation causes blindness (Wrong! We would have a lot of blind people out there...). Other myths include Kellogg's cornflakes will help you stop masturbating (Mr. Kellogg himself used to promote this idea... but he was antisex) and if you masturbate you will grow hair on the back of your hands (another crazy idea).

I mean, why did you hear me say the word masturbation and immediately feel the need to lighten the mood and tell a joke? You've got to ask yourself why you are uncomfortable with the topic? You, who wanted to write a book on vaginas?

LL: Yowza. Good question. I discovered my vagina at a young age, and I spent years masturbating and thinking I was doing something wrong.

CG: When children do this at such a young age, I prefer to call it *discovery*—the pressing down on the labia and the mons pubis, which then stimulates the clitoral shaft. Lots of girls do it all the time. I like to differentiate between this and inserting your finger into your vagina or stimulating your clitoris directly...though all of it is completely normal and part of this chapter, so we can lump it all together. There is a lot of variability when it comes to girls masturbating. Some young girls can go on a rocking horse or a real horse to get stimulated. Others rub their mons against something hard like a bedpost. Others stimulate different parts of their genitalia. But I interrupted you, please go on with what you were saying.

LL: So I "discovered" myself all the time! That sounds silly. It sounds like a legal term, like when a lawyer is "in a period of discovery"! Anyway, it felt so, so good. Even though my parents never said a word to me, I *know* they had to have noticed, just like I occasionally notice or hear about my friend's daughters doing this out and about in their houses. But even though I never really got a negative message about it, I still thought I was doing something wrong. I remember hoping to myself that somehow it was "genetic." And I remember praying silently and hoping it was not my fault that I was doing this, but some kind of internal drive, which it was, but I never asked anyone at that age...and no one volunteered any information about it, either.

I also remember year after year after year making New Year's resolutions that I wouldn't "do that" anymore. And that was all before I was ten years old, and I didn't even have a name for it! All I knew is that it felt good, and I tried to stop, but the pleasure overcame me, and I didn't stop. So somehow, somewhere I thought it was wrong, though my parents never said a thing.

CG: They probably didn't know what to say. They probably even thought they were doing the right thing by not saying anything.

LL: I do remember vividly that my brother Brian said something to me. He was two years younger, and I must have been around ten, so he would have been eight. One night I asked him if I could watch TV in his room, he was watching some show, and he said, "Not if you touch your vagina." That was the first reference anyone made to me about my masturbating—discovering. At the time, I had thought he never even noticed. Kids can be so clueless, and I was *definitely* clueless. But he obviously did notice, and I guess it bothered him. Or at least it bothered him that I was doing it in his presence. So after that I took it behind closed doors.

CG: How awkward.

LL: Not nearly as awkward as the other time I remember so vividly. It makes me want to cringe just thinking about it. My dad was president of a community college when I was growing up. At the time this memory happened I must have been around nine. My mom was back in school to get her college degree.

In those years my mom was in school a lot, so we spent more time at my dad's office. One day I was in his office, and he had a meeting down the hall. I was watching this small TV he had in his office while lying down on the floor. One thing led to another, and I started pressing on my vagina—you know, discovering—and I heard a noise behind me. It was my father's dean—Dean Young (not his real name)—standing there staring at me. In retrospect, he probably had that look of "*Oh, no—I was not supposed to see this—how do I back out of here without her noticing?*" But I *did* notice. I was mortified, and that vision was with me, torturing me, for years. Even last year, when I went back to New York for the fortieth anniversary of my father's being president of his community college, and I saw Dean Young—who had moved on to become president of his own community college twenty years prior—I thought to myself, "I wonder if he remembers that?"

CG: I guess it can be surprising to walk in on someone discovering, even if that person is a child.

LL: Or especially if she is a child. Now that I have my own kids, I see their natural curiosity about their own bodies, and I see them explore, like the time my son was three and was hitting his penis, and he said to me "Look, Mommy! I can make it stand up!" It is one of those experiences that remind you that these things are completely normal. One of my best friends has a daughter who does the same thing as I did, discovering her vagina, and she does it all over the house, too. My friend has gently told her to touch her private parts in her room, but she is completely unselfconscious, as many prepubescent girls are, and she does it all over, when she is in the living room watching a movie, in her room reading, in the car. It feels good, so she does it.

> An important take-home message here is that masturbation is completely normal, for adults and for children, but it is something that should be done privately, just like going to the bathroom.

CG: Can I chime in here? I raised boys, and you know I am so open and so easygoing, but I don't remember anything like this. I don't have these stories. But I do have stories of women coming to me with problems with their pelvic floor or an inability to orgasm, and as I work with them, I take their social history and hear all kinds of stories about feelings of shame and discomfort when it came to anything sexual. They have years and years, and layers and layers of negative messages to overcome.

LL: That is really sad.

CG: It is. Especially because masturbation is so good for you. For one thing, some women find it incredibly relaxing, and there is so much stress released after having an orgasm. And I will venture to bet that women need that after long days raising kids or at the office. Whatever women do, they are often overworked, racked with guilt (emotional energy), and exhausted, and masturbation can take the edge off. Though for some women masturbation is just about the furthest thing from relaxation.

Besides being healthy what is so valuable about masturbation is that it allows women to understand their own sexual response. Betty Dodson, PhD, a pioneer sex therapist and educator, said: [67]

---

[67] Stewart, *V Book: A Doctor's Guide to Complete Vulvovaginal Health,* 121.

"Masturbation is a way for all of us to learn about sexual response. It's an opportunity for us to explore our bodies and minds for all those sexual secrets we've been taught to hide, even from ourselves. What better way to learn about pleasure and being sexually creative? We don't have to perform or meet anyone else's standards, to satisfy the needs of a partner, or to fear criticism or rejection for failure. Sexual skills are like any other skills; they're not magically inherited, they have to be learned."

LL: I love that.

CG: Until recently our culture has not been ready to talk about masturbation openly. Well, maybe male masturbation because there have always been tons of jokes about that in the mainstream media and everyone seems to know and accept that males just…masturbate.

But female masturbation has always had this stigma and denial, which is why I am so thrilled to see it a drop more in the mainstream recently. Not that we are there yet, but I do sense that we are heading in that direction. The United States, especially New England, was deeply influenced by Puritan beliefs and culture, and we still feel some of that influence today. The Puritans had left England in 1620 because they felt that the church there was too lenient and accepting. Puritans were not very open-minded and accepting. The man was ruler over his wife, and if the kids were undisciplined, it was seen as a sin. And sexuality was completely taboo. There was no talk of sex, no having sex for fun, and sex was only for procreation. Americans have changed a lot since then, but we still have vestigial values we can trace back to that period.

LL: I guess back then when one in ten women died in childbirth, and there was no reliable contraception that certainly put a damper on interest in sex.

I was really curious about this idea a few months ago, and I discovered a book on GoodReads, which really hit this point home. *The Weaker Vessel*[68], by Lady Antonia Fraser, shows the details of women's lives in the seventeenth century, and it was not pretty. Women had very few rights and were not seen as equal to men—in fact at one point the belief was that the sperm contained a teeny baby. The mother was simply a vessel. On old headstones the father's name is often given but not the mother's for that reason.

Reading that book was fascinating, but it also made me very thankful to be living in this time period. Women live much longer now thanks to modern

---

68 Fraser, Antonia, *The Weaker Vessel: Women's Lot in Seventeenth-Century England* (London: Phoenix, 1984).

medicine, and the quality of our lives is better thanks to contraception. As a result women can have intercourse for pleasure and also without risk of pregnancy—or death.

CG: Our culture and attitudes toward sexuality, as well as our willingness to participate in sexuality, has changed tremendously in the past one hundred years as a result of these changes. Now that we don't have the fears we once had about death and pregnancy, what is stopping us from enjoying sexuality and seeing it as a gift? We still have our hang-ups, and we still have a long way to go. I think that many other cultures in many other countries are way ahead of us in this arena, and so much cross-culturalism has had a big impact on us just relaxing more.

LL: Plus the younger generations are just so much more likely to be open to new ideas, and they are likely to think it is not such a big deal to talk about masturbation. Why is it that the younger generations are always more open to change?

CG: All that being said, masturbation was not something that could be spoken about publicly even as recently as 1994. At that time, Dr. Jocelyn Elders, an amazing and progressive woman, was named the fifteenth surgeon general of the United States by President Bill Clinton. Dr. Elders was very progressive, as doctors and public health advocates often are. She did a few controversial things. But her downfall was making a public comment about masturbation. In 1994 Dr. Elders was invited to speak at a United Nations conference on AIDS. She was asked whether it would be appropriate to promote masturbation as a means of preventing young people from engaging in riskier forms of sexual activity. She replied, "I think that it is part of human sexuality, and perhaps it should be taught." Well, DUH! *Of course* this is true, and of course she was right. Dr. Elders—you go, girl. But this one remark caused a great deal of controversy and caused her to lose the support of the White House (that is, she was asked to step down).

LL: No doubt there was some poll somewhere showing that Americans thought this was terrible, and President Clinton just could not keep on supporting her because that would risk his approval numbers going down.

CG: It's all about those numbers in politics, isn't it?

LL: Amen.

CG: Anyway, the point is that as recently as 1994, not even twenty years ago, Americans could not accept masturbation. Well, baby, the times they are a-changing. And Dr. Elders, this chapter is dedicated to you.

> **TOP TEN REASONS TO MASTURBATE**
>
> 1. Masturbation is good for you. There are lots of health benefits!
> 2. If you are craving a "quickie," but don't want to make a big mess in your bed.
> 3. If you don't have a partner, you can still have a satisfying sexual experience.
> 4. If your partner is away or sleeping, you can still have an orgasm.
> 5. It helps you discover what you like, including how to have an orgasm. You can experiment with fantasies, vibrators, stimulating your clitoris or vagina in different ways—and then you can share this information with your partner.
> 6. For a quick pick-me-up
> 7. It helps relax your body right before you get to bed, and it helps you sleep better.
> 8. You don't have to worry about getting pregnant
> 9. You don't have to worry about sexually transmitted infections (STIs)
> 10. If you fall asleep in the middle of masturbating, your "partner" won't feel insulted!

LL: So what if some women readers aren't comfortable with masturbating or they don't know how or don't know where to start? But now that they know about the health and other benefits they want to give it a try, or at least get more experience with it?

CG: There are lots of great books out there. There are even great websites and YouTube videos that will show you how. But of course, if you do a search on that, you'll probably find a lot of porn! Maybe you can preview some sites and put some ideas in the Suggested Resources at the end of this chapter.

There is a lot out there about masturbation in general.

LL: Do you have any recommendations for where to start?

CG: Yes. The woman who was a pioneer in this field, Betty Dodson, wrote a great book called *Sex for One*. I would start there.

LL: All right. On to our next topic. But just before we move on, a word about vibrators.

VIBRATORS

There are many ways to masturbate, but the two most common ways are using fingers and vibrators. Vibrators are used to stimulate a woman's vagina and clitoris; they can be used solo or with a partner.

Use of vibrators is very common. More than half of 2,056 women, aged eighteen to sixty, used a vibrator either during masturbation or intercourse, says Debby Herbenick, PhD, MPH, associate director of the Center for Sexual Health Promotion at Indiana University, Bloomington.[69]

Vibrators were first invented in the late 1800s and quickly became popular. They were even sold in the Sears Roebuck catalog. But because they appeared to be connected to porn, they dropped off the mainstream retail market in the 1920s. Vibrators became more popular during the sexual revolution of the 1960s. In recent years, they have become more visible in mainstream culture, with the most notable example of this being a discussion about vibrators on the HBO show *Sex and the City*.

Today they are so popular that when you do a search on Amazon.com for vibrators, there are over 35,000 results!

There are many different styles of vibrators. There are clitoral stimulators, dildo-shaped vibrators (shaped like a penis), and rabbit-style ones that can go inside your vagina and stimulate your clitoris at the same time (this was the kind they liked on *Sex and the City*). There are literally hundreds of different styles.

---

[69] Herbenick, Debby, Michael Reece, Stephanie Sanders, Brian Dodge, Annahita Ghassemi, and J. Dennis Fortenberry, "Prevalence and Characteristics of Vibrator Use by Women in the United States: Results from a Nationally Representative Study," *Journal of Sexual Medicine*, 6, 7 (2009) : 1857–1866.

> *Redbook* magazine tried to make it easier for readers to choose a vibrator by having readers review them—check out this link: http://www.redbookmag.com/love-sex/advice/vibrator-reviews.
>
> Some sex therapists warn that too much use of vibrators can make a woman less likely to orgasm with a partner. When possible it is important for partners to learn how to arouse and stimulate each other. A vibrator may become a crutch for some people and this may prevent the normal experimentation experienced by partners. But just as with everything else, everything in moderation.

Suggested Resources:

Barbach, Lonnie, *For Yourself: The Fulfillment of Female Sexuality* (New York: Signet, 2000).

Chudnofsky, Lisa, "Your Hands-on Guide to Solo Sex," *Cosmopolitan*. n.d. http://www.cosmopolitan.com/sex-love/tips-moves/solo-sex.

Dodson, Betty, *Sex for One: The Joy of Selfloving* (New York: Three Rivers Press, 1996).

Fetters, K. Aleisha, "The 7 Best Masturbation Tips," *Women's Health*, n.d. http://www.womenshealthmag.com/sex-and-relationships/masturbation-tips.

Funny YouTube video! http://www.youtube.com/watch?v=1GyUwAq88A0.

CHAPTER 14

Fantasy and Your Biggest Sex Organ—Your Brain

Definition of Fantasy

LL: OK, I have to admit, I had a very different idea of how I wanted this chapter to go before *Fifty Shades of Grey* got so popular. I mean, I can't even think about fantasy now without thinking of that book. Part of me just doesn't get why it's so popular…and part of me totally gets it.

CG: The best place to start when talking about fantasies — *Fifty Shades* or not — is just with defining the terms. I mean, what is fantasy?

Most women would agree that a lot of sexuality takes place in your mind, not just in your body or erogenous spots or genital area. Or at the least it starts in your brain and there is a lot of communication between your brain and your body. If your body wants sex but your mind is not on board, then it is very hard to relax and enjoy and be sexual. Same thing if your mind is in the mood but your body is not responding, maybe it's tired or sick or has some sort of health issue. Both body and mind have to be on board. It's symbiotic.

Also, when I say *brain* I don't mean the physical cells that are inside your skull. I really mean your mind—where your thoughts reside.

And sexually speaking, there are two different kinds of thoughts going on in your mind that we need to differentiate between—there are <u>sexual thoughts</u> like

"Ooh, that guy is hot. I love just watching his pecs...I wonder what he would be like in bed?" or

"It felt so amazing the last time I had oral sex...I wonder if we can recreate that scene?" or even

"The kids are finally in bed, and we haven't had sex in a week...oh, I could really use fifteen extra minutes of sleep, but we haven't had sex for so long so I'm gonna 'get' in the mood..."

These sexual thoughts make you feel good and usually help you get aroused. When your mind starts thinking some of these thoughts, then your body often follows... physiological changes occur, like your vulva gets engorged, and your vagina starts to lubricate. A woman may have a heightened sense of touch. Her body may feel tingly, and she may feel a fluttering below her stomach. Women can sometimes make their bodies feel this way and get into the mood just by thinking sexual thoughts. Women often turn themselves on, and we can do that whether or not someone else is around or available.

And then there are *fantasies*, which are more like stories or narratives in a woman's brain. In *Getting the Sex You Want*,[70] author Tammy Nelson writes about our "erotic imagination." She defines this as including curiosity (anything you are curious about, even if you don't want to do anything about it), fantasy (anything you think about), and action (what you actually do).

Women can use either fantasies or sexual thoughts to get themselves turned on. Sexual thoughts alone may not do it for you, and you may need a fantasy. Or

---

[70] Nelson, Tammy, *Getting the Sex You Want: Shed Your Inhibitions and Reach New Heights* (Quiver Kindle, 2008).

maybe you need a fantasy to have an orgasm. Everyone is different, and all our bodies react differently to different thoughts and different kinds of touches.

A woman also may like to share her fantasy with her partner. Or, as in *Fifty Shades of Grey*, her partner might want to share a fantasy with her. The two of them can role-play or act out the fantasy. Some women are into that and some are not. Some enjoy it for its own sake, and some use it as a way to make things more interesting and exciting. Elle magazine and MSNBC did an online survey of over seventy-seven thousand adults, and when asked "What have you done to spice up your sex life in the last year?" one-third (34 percent) said they had talked about or acted out sexual fantasies.[71]

What have you done to spice up your sex life in the last year?[72] Sixty-four percent of respondents said they used massage, 59 percent bathed together, 59 percent used lingerie, 54 percent tried a new sexual position, 41 percent went on a romantic getaway, 40 percent used a vibrator, 37 percent watched porn, 34 percent talked about or acted out sexual fantasies, 23 percent had anal sex, 22 percent had sex in public, 21 percent integrated food into sex (e.g., chocolate sauce, whipped cream), 18 percent tried light S&M (e.g., restraints, spanking), 14 percent videotaped themselves having sex or posed for pictures in the nude, and 5 percent engaged in a threesome.

LL: Some of those statistics seem very high to me.

CG: Just like any survey you need to look at it in more detail. My guess is that this audience—readers of Elle, women who are going online to answer a survey on sex, and women who are willing to openly discuss their sex lives—tend to skew a bit younger. But their sample size was very large so we do know that a lot of women are doing a lot to spice up their sex lives, even if these results do skew younger.

Both sexual thoughts and fantasies stem from a woman's mind, and they work very well with her body to help her feel aroused and feel sexual. Because they both stem from your mind (or brain), you will often hear that "a woman's biggest sex organ is her brain."

LL: I remember hearing that when I was a teenager, and I was just starting to have sexual thoughts. That statement hit me as *so* true.

---

[71] "What You Said When We Asked About Sex," *MSN*, n.d., accessed September 2012, http://www.msnbc.msn.com/id/12410076/ns/health-sexual_health/t/what-you-said-when-we-asked-about-sex/.
[72] Ibid.

CG: If a woman is happy with the partner she is with and being physical with, if she is having some kind of sexual thoughts or fantasies or she is just enjoying the feeling of being physical with her partner, then the stars are truly aligned.

LL: I know a lot of women like to talk about their sexual fantasies with their partners, but that is one thing I like to keep to myself—up in my brain and stuck there.

CG: That is fine, you who are writing a book on vaginas and seem to be open about everything else. No, seriously, a lot of women have a lot of contradictory ideas about sex, and it comes down to whatever works for you. So in thirteen years of marriage you haven't shared your fantasies with your husband?

LL: Nope. It's almost like I am scared I will jinx them. They work so well to help me to have an orgasm, so I don't want to do anything to disturb the balance of things. Besides, I just read this awesome blog by individual and couples counselor and prolific blogger Julie Jeske, and she said to "embrace your sexual dichotomies."[73] So I am!

CG: Well, as I always say, to each her own, just as different women get aroused by different kinds of fantasies. Some like the spanking and S&M type of fantasies like in *Fifty Shades*. Others like the "being carried away into the sunset" fantasies, and still others like the dominatrix fantasies where they are in control, and their partner needs to submit to them. A lot of fantasies are about control and power on some level. And by the way, we know that this is appealing to a lot of women—at least reading about it—because it really sells! Just like *Fifty Shades of Grey*, romance novels of all kinds are over a billion-dollar-per-year business, and this genre of fiction sells more copies of books than any other.

I read this great book called *Why Women Have Sex*[74] by Cindy Meston and David Buss, researchers at the University of Texas at Austin. In this book they analyze why so many women have fantasies about power and control, and they point out that "In many erotic romance novels, the hero uses some measure of physical force, "taking" the heroine sexually, despite her protestations and resistance..."

LL: All right, I am already uncomfortable with this concept...do we have to go on?

CG: Listen! You will like the ending, so just continue listening.

---

[73] "Embrace Your Sexual Dichotomies," Julie Jeske (blog), Accessed January 11, 2013, http://www.juliejeske.com/2012/04/.

[74] Meston, Cindy M. and David M. Buss, *Why Women Have Sex: Understanding Sexual Motivations from Adventure to Revenge (and Everything in Between)* (New York: Times Books, 2009).

"A few psychologists argue that because some women find these forceful sexual submission depictions to be arousing, they reflect psychological pathology or socially internalized gender scripts that urge women to link sex with submission to men. *The actual scientific evidence, however,* supports a different interpretation. Psychologist Patricia Hawley studied forceful sexual submission fantasies in a sample of nearly nine hundred women. She found that women who tended to have and enjoy these sexual force fantasies, far from being submissive or pathological, in fact were more dominant, more independent, and higher in self-esteem than other women. Women who were less socially powerful had fewer sexual fantasies in which they were forced to sexually submit."[75]

Talk about sexual dichotomies!

Choosing the fantasies that are right for you

CG: Many women have go-to fantasies to get them in the mood and keep them there. And some women still don't know exactly what turns them on. Also, what might have turned on a woman when she was younger may not do the trick as she gets a bit older. In particular, perimenopause or menopause sometimes causes your sex drive and your hormones to change, so you may need to figure out what you like again. But if a woman has not yet discovered what she likes, any time is a good time to start.

LL: I LOVE the quote from Regena Thomashauer that I read in Dr. Lissa Rankin's book *What's Up Down There*[76]:

"Most women don't know what turns us on. How could we? It's not like our moms pulled us onto their knees and said "Puberty is coming, so we're gonna learn what turns you on." And you can't leave it up to your boyfriend. Guys don't know what turns on a woman.

That's why I write and teach what I do—to educate women about how to begin to learn about their relationship to pleasure. If you don't know what pleasures you, you'll never get in touch with your desires. Take the time to learn the difference between what it feels like to touch the palm of your hand, how it feels to run your fingers across your belly or down the

---

75 Meston and Buss, *Why Women Have Sex: Understanding Sexual Motivations from Adventure to Revenge (and Everything in Between)*, 207.
76 Rankin, *What's Up Down There? Questions You'd Only Ask Your Gynecologist If She Was Your Best Friend*, 84-85, quoting Regena Thomashauer, Sister Goddess, author, and founder of Mama Gena's School of Womanly Arts.

inside of your thigh. What parts of your [vulva] feel good? What pressures do you enjoy? Without learning, how can you allow your lover to gratify you?

There's a scene in the Julia Roberts movie *Runaway Bride* where someone asks her what kinds of eggs she likes, but she doesn't know. When she dated a guy who liked scrambled eggs, she ate scrambled eggs. When he liked fried eggs, she ate hers fried. When he liked hard-boiled, she ate hard-boiled. In one scene, she finally lines them up and tastes them all, so she can make a decision, independent of any man.

A woman can definitely be seduced into running that kind of experiment with her own body. Taste. Touch. Experiment. Discover."

CG: That is a great quote. This is great advice for physically getting to know your body and also getting to know what fantasies turn you on.

So when it comes down to fantasies, if you know what you like and it works for you, great. If you don't have a good arsenal of fantasies and you need some, here are some suggestions from fantasies I read about on the Internet:

Need a little help getting your fantasy life going? Here is a menu of different fantasies that other women like[77]. Try one out or use your imagination to think of a new one. And remember, fantasy comes from relaxing and letting your mind wander.

1. Sexual Submission

After a long day in the office and hours of helping the kids with homework and bedtime routines many women turn to fantasies about sexual submission. Perhaps after all of the decisions we need to make, it is enjoyable to be controlled or even "forced" to do something sexual. Perhaps someone forces you to wear a see-through dress, your nipples are hardened, you are blindfolded…Or maybe it is just plain fun to imagine a stranger, or someone powerful having his way with you sexually. It worked for Anastasia Steele in *Fifty Shades of Grey*…we dare you to try it out, too (or just imagine it).

---

[77] These fantasy ideas were taken from a number of different websites on the Internet. There are thousands of fantasies out there, but the ones listed below were repeated over and over again, and we thought they would be the most relatable.

2. Voyeuristic Sex

Your lover ravishes you and invites his friends, or your friends, to watch. Or you seduce your partner in a public place—on a beach, in a parking lot, where you know you will be "caught in the act." Or maybe *you* are the one who spies on someone else having sex. Anyone you know or even a complete stranger can be the subject of this fantasy. You would be mortified if anyone ever found out. But that's exactly what makes it so delicious. You know they are watching your every move, but you groan anyway because you can't help it.

3. Three's Company

Or maybe even four or five or a whole room full of people. It could be you and your partner and another man. Or you and your partner and another woman. Or a room full of total strangers whom you will never see again. You feel all four hands on your body, touching so many places at once…

4. Celebrity Sex

You luck out and get a ticket to the Academy Awards and then George Clooney (or replace any other celebrity name) catches your eye, and you share a flirtatious moment. One thing leads to another and you are whisked off in his limo. Or in another scenario you are home on a Friday night after a long week at work. Your husband is flying in on a red-eye and will be home in the morning. Matthew McConaughey knocks on your door, somehow sensing you were home. He brings flowers and dinner. You share a wild night and send him on his way before the sun comes up.

5. Romance Is Alive and Well

Imagine your perfect, ideal partner courting you and seducing you. He treats you like you have never been treated before. He pampers you and worships the ground you walk on. And he understands you without you having to explain anything to him. His one wish is to please you both in and out of bed.

6. Mile High Club

You're in an airplane taking your first vacation with a new partner. You have heard about people having sex in bathrooms on airplanes but never in a million years thought you would be one of them. But your partner suggests the idea, and the next thing you know you are hot and heavy and not listening when the captain says to fasten your seatbelt.

7. Sex with a Stranger

Imagine walking down the street and catching someone's eye. You feel a sense of attraction like you have never felt before. You both look away and then turn back at the same time. You don't know his name or where he lives or how old he is, but the next thing you know you are in each other's arms in an alleyway. You spend the next hour doing things you have never imagined (using condoms of course) and then you leave, completely exhausted but exhilarated.

8. Naughty Schoolgirl

You are in an all-girls school in England in the year 1800. You are living on the estate of an earl who cares first and foremost about obedience. But you are a naughty, mischievous, fifteen-year-old schoolgirl, and you are always being spanked by the headmaster. He calls you into his office and this time he has a gleam in his eye. He takes out a paddle and tells you to pull up your skirt. You count to ten and after each paddling say, "Thank you sir, may I please have another?" After each spanking his hands get closer and closer to your clitoris and your nipples.

9. Good girls Gone "Bad"

All your life you have followed the rules. You don't speed, litter, or have casual sex. But then you go through a major change — either you go through a really tough time or you just decide that you are tired of being *good* all the time. You decide to go to a strip club and join the dancers out on the floor. Or you seduce someone you have had your eyes on for a long time. You do whatever you want without any feelings of remorse or shame and you make no apologies.

10. Taking Control

You have always been the one to follow someone else's lead, but now you want to take control. You tie up your lover while he is asleep and turn him into your sex slave. You tell him exactly what you want, and you punish him if he does not follow your orders.

11. Sex with an Ex

You go to the grocery store on a Saturday night, and who is there by himself but your ex. One thing leads to another, the groceries are abandoned, and you are on your way to his place. The familiar smells and feelings are both comfortable and erotic. You might have made a terrible long-term couple, but the short-term sex is all you care about right now.

12. Girl-on-Girl

It's you and the woman of your dreams. Your woman of choice could be a celebrity like JLo or the woman who works down the hall. It could be a nameless, faceless woman or a friend from high school. Whoever she is imagine your bodies entwined. Explore every part of her. Whether you are naturally attracted to women or both men and women or just men, let go of any thoughts of reality and let the fantasy arouse you.

13. Anything-Taboo Sex

No one ever has to know about what you think about in the deepest part of your imagination. So let it all out — into your imagination — anything taboo, your deepest desires that arouse you. It's erotic, exhilarating, and completely taboo. Remember that fantasy by definition is just that — and you never have to tell a soul.

The Importance of Fantasy in a Relationship

CG: Here is some homework — try out these (or any other fantasies) and see which ones make you feel the most sexually aroused. First think about them. Let them marinate in your brain and close your eyes and see which one or ones help you to feel excited.

Also, if a woman wants to share her fantasy with her partner, or if she wants to act it out, she should take small steps, make sure she feels safe, and then *try it out*. Perhaps start with something simple like sharing "I like it when you take all of my clothes off" and judge his reaction. If she feels too shy or embarrassed or even ashamed to talk about her fantasy, she should ask herself if she thinks her partner will be open to hearing it. Her partner should listen kindly and be positive about any of her fantasies. Whether a woman and her partner want to try the fantasy out is up to them.

LL: A lot of women feel a lot of shame over their sexual thoughts and fantasies, so it might be difficult for them to broach the subject. Also, what if a woman is shy and hasn't done this before? What would you recommend?

CG: Well, I think there is a lot to be said about shame. Let's talk about that next. For some women it is not really shame but exposure. When they say their fantasies out loud, they can feel exposed or vulnerable. But if a woman wants to share her sexual thoughts and fantasies, here are a few ideas for how to bring them up.

- The next time you are in bed with your partner and there is some peace and quiet, tell your partner that you want to share a fantasy with him. Ask him to just listen and not necessarily try the fantasy out at that moment. Explain that perhaps at some point in the future…if one thing leads to another, you could explore the fantasy. If not, then your partner will likely let it marinate and perhaps fantasize about it, too, before you both try it out.
- Write your partner a love note that details the fantasy or fantasies you have been thinking about. Suggest that you try one or all of these out the next time you get a chance.
- The next time you both have some quiet time together tell your partner that you have been wanting to talk about this fantasy and have not known how to bring it up. This doesn't have to be while you're in bed. You could be in the car on your way to dinner. Maybe play a game where you give clues, and your partner needs to guess the details of your fantasy.
- Start slowly by sharing a simple, safe fantasy, and not your most risqué one. For example tell him you like when he takes your clothes off slowly.
- Instead of telling your partner, use nonverbal language and *show* your partner what your fantasy is.
- Ask your partner to tell you his or her fantasies that you have never heard about before.

Fantasies can be a wonderful and creative way of keeping passion alive in a relationship. Or they can be a way to just have fun.

Fantasy and Your Biggest Sex Organ—Your Brain

It's also important for everyone to know that:

- Fantasizing does not mean that you are dissatisfied with your partner or with your sexual life.
- Just because you *think* it does not mean that you necessarily would want it in real life.
- Just because you are curious about it does not mean anything bad or harmful.
- Just because you fantasize about something may not mean you want to act it out. Or maybe it does. You get to decide whether or not fantasy becomes reality.
- Reality and fantasy are two different experiences. In fantasy all of the experiences are exactly right because you control them. Reality is hard to control! For example you may fantasize about having sex in the water but then when you do you may notice that your lubrication rinses away.
- If you do communicate your fantasies to your partner, then you may want to fill him/her in on the above facts as well.

Many women are happily married or in committed relationships and still fantasize about someone else, often a nameless, faceless person or it could even be their friend's husband or their husband's friend or a woman who lives in their apartment complex or someone they met while working out. Often this also comes out in their dreams. They wake up realizing they were dreaming about having sex with another man. *Can it* indicate something is wrong in your relationship? Sure it can—and I think women need to explore this—but often it is just fantasy. All of this is typical and all of it is normal. It becomes a problem when a woman turns a fantasy into reality and cheats on her partner, or less commonly, when a woman becomes so obsessed with a fantasy that she has a hard time enjoying her reality.

It is also completely normal and natural for some heterosexual women to fantasize about having sex with women or watching other men have sex with other women. Many heterosexual women have sexual dreams about other women. This is completely natural. Some women choose to explore whether or not it means they may be bisexual or lesbian, but in more cases than not they are heterosexual women who have fluid fantasies that never play out in their lives.

LL: That reminds me of something I have been worried about before. I have had lesbian dreams before and also fantasies that involve both men and women. I definitely consider myself heterosexual, but there was a period in time when I did question this. I was in graduate school getting my master's in counseling, and I was taking a class called Counseling Sexual Minorities, which was taught by my favorite professor. A couple months into the class, I got what I now realize was like medical school syndrome — where every time first-year medical students study a different syndrome, they think they have it! So I was putting some pieces together — I had experienced occasional lesbian dreams since I was a child, some of my fantasies included other women… maybe I was a lesbian!

CG: So what did you do?

LL: Well, first I told my husband. And he was great, which relieved me. He said if I wanted to explore, he was OK with that — then he got a twinkle in his eye and added the oh-so-typical male response, "But can I watch?"

The next class I went to, I could not stop thinking about it. In the middle of the seminar, we had a break, and I pulled my professor aside and told her what I was thinking. She asked me if I felt attracted to women in real life, and I said no, and she smiled, then laughed, and said, "I have heterosexual dreams, and believe me, I am not heterosexual!" This one comment made me realize on a gut level that maybe we are just fluid when it comes to our sexuality. And it also confirmed to me that sometimes a fantasy is just a fantasy.

Getting rid of any lingering shame or embarrassment
CG: It is so great that your husband and your professor were both so supportive and nonjudgmental. And that probably helped you to figure out what was going on with you. Everyone has periods of questioning, and not just about their sexuality but about their worth, their talent, their looks, their intelligence. If you are surrounded by supportive and nonjudgmental people, you tend to experience less shame and embarrassment.

Sometimes fantasies cause women to feel embarrassed or ashamed. Sometimes they have the fantasy anyway and then go on and feel badly about themselves. And other times they suppress the fantasy. I know from my experience with numerous patients that there are a lot of women who feel some sense of shame or embarrassment over something sexual, whether it is a fantasy they have or more often a past embarrassing experience. Maybe it is a *cringeworthy* moment from the past — like when one patient's ex-husband said she was boring in bed, or when another let out a lot of gas while having sex with a fairly new partner. Or it could be about something more ongoing, like one of my patients who had a great deal of shame about her body and appearance. Other women have shame or embarrassment over the look or feel or smell of their vagina, their weight…really anything that makes her feel bad.

As you can see from the guided meditation we did earlier, there is so, so much that goes into what happens behind the scenes in your brain—both consciously and subconsciously. There are years and years and layers and layers of messages. There are your past experiences, your parents' past experiences, and those of your siblings and friends and even your friends' friends.

Shame is a really awful-feeling emotion. It's embarrassing, and the more we feel it, the more we want to hide it and bury it. But the problem with that is that, as with anything else, the more you try to bury a feeling, the bigger it gets. *The more you try to hide your shame and embarrassment, the more it can harm you.* It sometimes manifests itself as a physical illness. It has even been linked to depression.[78]

LL: I need to restate that *part of this revolution MUST include a commitment for women everywhere to confront and then to get rid of their lingering shame and embarrassment*. Just as it is time to accept our vaginas and let them come out of the closet, so it is time to release any negative feelings about our fantasies or sexual thoughts and let them come out of the closet. Not that you have to tell anyone your cringeworthy moments to make this happen (though it may help), but it is time to drop the feelings of shame and embarrassment that surround these thoughts. They serve no positive purpose, and they are harmful to your health.

Some women are *taught* and *encouraged* to feel ashamed of their sexual organs, their sexuality, their sexual desires (or lack of desire), their sexual experience (or inexperience), and so on. So often these thoughts get stuck in our heads, and they overshadow our thoughts and diminish our joy. This is counterproductive. Enough is enough already. If we are having a revolution here, we should free ourselves from the evil tyrants—our brains.

---

[78] Kaufman, G., *The Psychology of Shame* (London: Routledge, 1993).

Join the Revolution! *Embrace Fantasy!*

The popularity of *Fifty Shades of Grey* shows that many women are enthusiastically embracing fantasy—though some may just be doing this on their Kindles.

To embrace fantasy we need to do the following:

(1) Say no to any leftover feelings of shame. Many women were taught to equate feelings of sexuality with shame. Many women feel some sort of shame when thinking about their own sexual body parts. Sometimes, our parents and our communities taught us this explicitly. Other times, we picked it up implicitly, as part of our culture. Just as "the last thing a fish would ever notice would be water," we breathe in and absorb the general thoughts, attitudes, values, and norms of the environment in which we live without thinking about them. It can be really hard to shake the habits we pick up from our environment—especially if we don't even recognize they exist. So to all of this shame we say "No! We will not feel shame over our sexuality any longer!"

(2) Enjoy sexual thoughts. If you enjoy having your earlobes sucked on or your toes licked, and it is something that you want to do…enjoy it. If you feel aroused by the idea of being blindfolded or dominated, then don't deny those thoughts, either.

(3) Want to feel aroused but you don't? Try out some fantasies and figure out which ones work for you. Reread some of the suggestions in this chapter or go online to find others.

(4) Don't feel badly if you fantasize about nameless, faceless people, or a young guy you saw at the gym, or a friend, or a woman if you are heterosexual or men if you are a lesbian. Don't worry if you have sex dreams about other people of any gender even if you are happily partnered. All of this is normal. If you want to turn one of these "forbidden" fantasies into reality, but you could hurt a relationship or another person by doing this, then first talk to a counselor or friend. They can help you examine your motivations and help you figure out how best to proceed. If the fantasy is just used as escapism and does not take over your life, then see it as exactly that, escapism.

> (5) Consider sharing your fantasies with a partner or trusted someone... or don't. The great thing about fantasies is that by definition they are in your head, and you can choose to keep them there or not.

LL: Remember Becky's triangle from the last chapter? It is relevant here, too. Basically, any time you want to change what is going on in your brain, you can use the triangle—or cognitive behavioral therapy—to help you. Feelings from the past can cause you to feel badly, and they can affect how you feel about your fantasy or sexuality. This in turn can make you feel less sexual and change your behavior—you might have or initiate less sex. Try this exercise below to get rid of the shame and embarrassment and cringeworthy moments and you can change your world!

> Join the Revolution! Free your brain. Get rid of your cringeworthy moments!
>
> How do we get rid of these awful moments? Here is a step-by-step guide.
>
> Caveat: if you are thinking about a moment that is too painful—like sexual abuse, rape, or anything else that causes extreme pain—stop here and do not do this alone. Ask a counselor or friend or spiritual leader to be there with you.
>
> 1. WRITE—Write down something that causes you shame or an awkward moment or moments from the past that cause you embarrassment when you think of them. Write the moment(s) down in your journal or on a blank piece of paper.
>
>   If you have more than one moment (and most of us do) just take one at a time—the easiest one first.
>
> 2. EMBRACE—After writing down the moment, think about it. Try to relive it in your mind. After you relive it in your mind, think about the feelings you are experiencing. It's OK if they are awful. Try to figure out where you "feel" it in your body—is it a queasy feeling in your stomach? Is it tightness in your chest?

> "Talk" to the feeling—the queasiness or the tightness—and tell it "it's OK, this happened in the past. Everyone has embarrassing moments." Use any other neutral messages you can give it. Embrace—almost try to *enjoy*—those awful feelings that came up when the experience was happening. This may feel painful and might make you cringe even more than before, but it is worth it—you are "owning" the feelings, and sometimes the feelings need to get worse before they get better.
>
> 3. LET GO—Advice from my mom. One thing she has shared with me over and over through the years is this advice. "Laura, forgive yourself" and "Laura, talk to yourself." Say out loud to yourself (in these words or make up your own) "Laura—boy, was that embarrassing, but you know what? I forgive you! That was so in the past! EVERYONE has moments like that, and I just have more of them, but you know what? Who cares! Life is so short—I can't stay in a safe shell like a turtle my whole life. And sometimes when I do things and stick my neck out, I get embarrassed, and you know what? Who cares! Life is too short to dwell."
>
> 4. Did it work? Maybe not right away but by bringing the uncomfortable emotions or buried thoughts to the surface, you are better able to work on them, dream about them, or talk about them to friends. And the more you do this, the more their importance diminishes, making you feel better and free from those emotions.

CG: The important thing here is that everyone is going to have bad times, sad times, and awkward times, but it is what you do with those moments that will have a lasting impact on your brain. It goes hand in hand with growing up, accepting these experiences, evolving, moving on…leaving these experiences where they should stay—in the past.

I suggest that women speak with a counselor, therapist, psychologist or anyone who can do talk therapy to help them get past thoughts that are inhibiting their lives. I also suggest they speak with their doctors about medication if their doctor thinks there is an underlying issue like depression or anxiety; as many as one out of every five women has one or more forms of anxiety or depression. But many women can help talk themselves through basic changes, and all women can learn to forgive themselves, get rid of the shame in their lives, and move on.

Suggested Resources:

Kahr, Brett, *Who's Been Sleeping in Your Head: The Secret World of Sexual Fantasies* (New York: Basic Books, 2009).

> Brett Kahr has studied the fantasy lives of thousands of people in Britain, and he has collected information about fantasies from 23,000 British and American men and women. One of the things he does in his book is report word for word what survey respondents fantasize about. It is absolutely fascinating—the range of responses, the wide variety of fantasies, the words the respondents choose to use when describing their fantasies!

Meston, Cindy M. and David M. Buss, *Why Women Have Sex: Understanding Sexual Motivations from Adventure to Revenge (and Everything in Between)* (New York: Times Books, 2009).

Nelson, Tammy, *Getting the Sex You Want: Shed Your Inhibitions and Reach New Heights* (Beverly, MA: Quiver, 2008).

A really great blog about sex and fantasy by Julie Jeske: http://www.juliejeske.com/.

CHAPTER 15

Orgasm

CG: This is one of my favorite topics. I could write a whole book on orgasms! Every woman is different (obviously) and feels good in different ways. Some women like having their hands held, others like having their feet rubbed. But orgasm seems to be the most talked about—sometimes obsessed about—part of feeling good and sexual.

LL: But now you're going to go into the whole thing about many women not being able to orgasm, right?

CG: Well, it is of interest. I see a lot of patients who have never had an orgasm and that is unfortunate. Some patients comment that they can only have an orgasm through touch, oral sex, or vibrators, and they feel inadequate that they do not have orgasm with penetration. Like we talked about before, the "Hollywood" image of "successful" sex, at least for heterosexual couples, is penis in vagina, thrusting, and the man and woman reach orgasm simultaneously.

LL: Well, that is true. But most women, myself included, don't always orgasm when having sex, and I really don't always feel the need to.

CG: And that is fine, of course. There *is never one correct definition of sex or intimacy or success*. The female orgasm is very complex, and it is unfortunate that some women have never had an orgasm. For most men, especially when they are young, it is easier to achieve orgasm.

LL: But isn't the bottom line on sex from a woman's perspective that they want the sex, have consensual sex, and then feel good afterward—both physically and psychologically? Orgasm or not?

CG: Yes. Yes, yes, yes. And I am probably reading way too much into this because of all that I have seen my patients go through—being raised by parents who made them feel that sex was "dirty." Or worse, incest or rape. So let me step back for a moment.

What is Orgasm?

CG: Orgasm is the climax, or the release of the sexual tension, that builds up during the initial stages of female arousal. Many researchers have tried to define and understand orgasm, and the understanding of sexual response in women has evolved over time. Different researchers have analyzed female sexual response in different ways and I will mention three common ways that have been discussed, from the older way of thinking about female sexual response to more current theories. Different descriptions will resonate more with some women than others. The more researchers can understand about female sexual response the more they will be able to help women understand how their bodies work, and thus help them to enhance their sexual experiences.

Orgasm: Linear Model

Masters and Johnson published a groundbreaking book in 1966 called *Human Sexual Response*[79]. In this book they described orgasm as the third phase of a four-phase cycle: arousal, plateau, orgasm, and resolution.

<u>Stage One: Arousal</u> A woman can be aroused by kissing, touch, smell, thoughts, movement, seeing erotic images, and taste, and when she feels aroused her nipples get erect, her breasts become fuller, and blood flows to her vulva. Blood vessels in her whole body will dilate and she may look flushed—sometimes this can be seen in her face or upper chest area. Lubrication comes through her vaginal walls. She might describe an engorged sensation in her genitals and that is partly because the erectile tissue in her genitals is standing up. The clitoral hood moves back, revealing more of the clitoris. Her heart rate and respiratory rate increase, as does her blood pressure.

<u>Stage Two: Plateau</u> The next stage involves a plateau. In the plateau stage the changes that happen in the arousal stage intensify. This is the stage right before orgasm and many women move back and forth between arousal and plateau. In the plateau stage the clitoris becomes more sensitive and withdraws slightly, sometimes retracting under the clitoral hood to avoid direct stimulation. In the plateau stage more lubrication is secreted.

<u>Stage Three: Orgasm</u> When a woman reaches orgasm it is often characterized as a full body experience. Women have rhythmic, involuntary contractions that are approximately 0.8 seconds apart. Women may feel the contractions in their uterus, anus, and vaginal muscles. The sensation of an orgasm can be compared to that of a sneeze in the way that it is a full release.

<u>Stage Four: Resolution</u> The last stage of sexual response is resolution. This is when a woman's body goes back to its normal state. Her heart rate goes back to normal and women may feel relaxed or fulfilled or even sleepy. Women may be stimulated again during this period to reach another orgasm, though only some women report having multiple orgasms.

I think that this is a good model and may resonate for some women, but not all women. This model was criticized by some researchers because it did not take into account some important factors like the place that sexuality and intimacy take inside relationships. Also this model was the same for both men and women and many health care professionals and researchers have found that sexual response is different for men and women. For example, women may move from sexual arousal to orgasm and satisfaction without experiencing

---

[79] Masters WH, Johnson VE. *Human Sexual Response*. Boston, MA: Little, Brown; 1966.

sexual desire, or they can experience desire, arousal, and satisfaction but not orgasm.[80]

Orgasm: Circular Model

The Circular Model is another model that may resonate with some women, but again probably not with all women. Sex educator and researcher Beverly Whipple improved upon the Linear Model and she wrote about this with Karen Brash-McGreer in 1997[81]. Whipple and Brash-McGreer proposed the idea that women have a circular sexual response and not a linear one. According to the Association of Reproductive Health Professionals[82]:

> "This concept is built on the Reed model, which comprises four stages: seduction (encompassing desire), sensations (excitement and plateau), surrender (orgasm), and reflection (resolution). By making Reed's model circular, Whipple and Brash-McGreer demonstrate that pleasant and satisfying sexual experiences may have a reinforcing effect on a woman, leading to the seduction phase of the next sexual experience. If, during reflection, the sexual experience did not provide pleasure and satisfaction, the woman may not have a desire to repeat the experience."

Whipple and Brash-McGreer explain that women may not experience all of the phases in the linear model. For example a woman may move from sexual arousal to orgasm to satisfaction without ever experiencing sexual desire. Or a woman can experience desire, arousal, and satisfaction, but not orgasm.

Orgasm: Non-linear Model

This is the most recent of the three models and I think the researchers were trying to find a theory that resonated with the women who could not relate as much to the previous two theories. Have you ever been lying in bed and your husband rolls over and expresses an interest in sex…sex is the last thing on your mind…but once

---

[80] Association of Reproductive Health Professionals, accessed January 2013, http://www.arhp.org/publications-and-resources/clinical-fact-sheets/female-sexual-response. Whipple B. Women's sexual pleasure and satisfaction. A new view of female sexual function. *The Female Patient* 2002;27:39-44.

[81] Whipple B, Brash-McGreer K. Management of female sexual dysfunction. In: Sipski ML, Alexander CJ, eds. *Sexual Function in People with Disability and Chronic Illness. A Health Professional's Guide.* Gaithersburg, MD: Aspen Publishers, Inc.; 1997, pp 509-534.

[82] http://www.arhp.org/publications-and-resources/clinical-fact-sheets/female-sexual-response, accessed January 2013.

you start kissing or becoming intimate you decide that this is actually a good thing? Dr. Rosemary Basson has built an entire theory around the simple idea that many women do not have a desire to initiate sex but once sex is initiated they enjoy it.

LL: Maybe this is why many moms tell their daughters not to say *no* to their partner (as long as they are feeling healthy and they are in a good relationship)? Because intimacy is important to a relationship. Women may not start out in the mood, especially if they are in a long-term relationship. But they may get in the mood and then once they are intimate they feel closer to their partners.

CG: Yes and this is in contrast to the first model we spoke about. The Linear Model starts with arousal but many women have sex for other reasons than because they feel aroused. Many of these women end up feeling aroused after they decide to have sex, but they decide to have sex for many other different reasons.

Sheryl Kingsburg and Gail Knudson wrote about this in *Psychiatry Weekly*[83]:

> Basson suggests that the linear model has a number of limitations, including: women often choose to be sexual for reasons other than sexual desire (eg, the desire to express love, to receive and share physical pleasure, to feel physical pleasure, to feel emotionally closer, to please a partner, and to increase one's own feelings of well-being); desire and arousal are difficult to disentangle as distinct entities; psychological motivation often overrides genital sensation; and women's sexual responses are variable from one occasion to another (noted that for many women a sexual encounter may begin without any desire initially present). Basson's model recognizes that female sexual functioning is more complex and is not as linear as male sexual functioning and many women initially begin a sexual encounter from a point of sexual neutrality. The decision to be sexual may come from a conscious wish for emotional closeness or as a result of seduction or suggestion from a partner. Women have many reasons for engaging in sexual activity other than simply sexual drive (i.e, sexual impulses that trigger sexual behavior).

> Sexual neutrality, or being receptive to (rather than initiating sexual activity), is considered a normal variation of female sexual functioning. In addition, women's arousal will often precede desire.

LL: You mentioned earlier that you think that some women will relate more to one model and some to another. Do you think that this is a result of age or stage in a relationship — in other words if a woman is in a new relationship she may

---

[83] S.A. Kingsburg and G. Knudson. Psychiatry Weekly, *Volume 6, Issue 4, February 14, 201*.

feel more initial desire but if she has been married for twenty years she may be more sexually neutral?

CG: I would never say that this is a rule—there are many women in long-term relationships who still feel that initial desire for example. But just like we have been saying all along that every woman is different and experiences things in different ways, I would say that this is true of female sexual response as well. In fact Kingsburg and Knudson cited a study that asked registered nurses which model of sexual response they most closely related to (they were given three models to choose from—the Masters and Johnson model, the Kaplan model which I do not explain here[84], and the Basson model) and approximately one-third endorsed the Masters and Johnson model, one-third endorsed Kaplan's model and one-third endorsed Basson's model. Of note, women with sexual concerns were more likely to endorse the Basson model.[85]

Clitoral and Vaginal Orgasms:

LL: I've heard something about different kinds of orgasm—one being better than the other—is there any truth to that? Why should it matter? Isn't an orgasm an orgasm?

CG: Through the years there has been much discussion about what defines a successful orgasm. In the past, there was delineation between two different kinds of orgasm—vaginal and clitoral. The thought was that there are two main ways that women can have an orgasm. A vaginal orgasm occurs when something is in the vagina, such as a penis, fingers, or a vibrator. That old brilliant but sometimes dead-wrong psychoanalyst Freud once said that this was the orgasm of the "physically adult woman," as opposed to the other kind of orgasms, which are called clitoral orgasms.

These ideas were perpetuated at a time before sexuality was truly studied, and they were usually written entirely from a male perspective. Later sexperts Alfred Kinsey and his team (as well as Masters and Johnson[86]) all found

---

84 For the sake of simplicity we will stick with the three main models, but note that Kaplan also made a significant contribution to this field in the early 1970's. The purpose of citing the Fisher study was to show that different women relate to different models of sexual response.

85 Sands M, Fisher MA. Women's endorsement of models of female sexual response: The nurses' sexuality study. *J Sex Med.* 2007;4:708-719.

86 William H. Masters and Virginia E. Johnson pioneered research into the nature of human sexual response and the diagnosis and treatment of sexual disorders and dysfunctions from 1957 until the 1990s. They observed couples in a laboratory setting and were able to debunk old myths about sexuality (for example, that vaginal lubrication during sex comes from the cervix) in addition to creating more successful methods of treating sexual disorders.

through interviews with thousands of women that most women do not in fact have vaginal orgasms. Since then, most experts have concluded that there is not a distinction between a vaginal or clitoral orgasm.

> **Frequency of Orgasm and Orgasm Statistics:**[87]
> The number one statistic to remember about female orgasms is that only 25 percent of women are consistently orgasmic during vaginal intercourse. This statistic comes from a comprehensive analysis of thirty-three studies that were done over the course of eighty years.[88]
>
> **If you are *HAPPY* with the frequency and type of orgasms you have, you are not alone!**
>
> …Among women currently in a partnered relationship, 62 percent say they are very satisfied with the frequency and consistency of their orgasms.[89]
>
> …About forty percent of both men and women said they were extremely pleased physically and extremely satisfied emotionally.[90]
>
> **If you are *UNHAPPY* with the frequency and type of orgasms you have, you are not alone!**
>
> …Between one-third and one-half of women experience orgasm infrequently and are dissatisfied with not being able to reach an orgasm more.[91]
>
> ---
>
> 87 Much of this research was collected by the Kinsey Institute and placed on their website (www.kinseyinstitute.org/). It is very interesting, and it is good research, but all research must be taken with a grain of salt, especially when it involves self-reported frequency of orgasm.
> 88 Lloyd, Elisabeth, *The Case of the Female Orgasm: Bias in the Science of Evolution* (Boston, MA: Harvard University Press, 2006).
> 89 Davis, C.M, J. Blank, L. Hung-Yu, and Consuelo Bonillas, "Characteristics of Vibrator Use Among Women," *Journal of Sex Research*, 33(4), 313-320.
> 90 Laumann, E., J.H. Gagnon, R.T. Michael, and S. Michaels, "The Social Organization of Sexuality: Sexual Practices in the United States" (Chicago, IL: University of Chicago Press, 1994). Also reported in the companion volume, Michael et al, *Sex in America: A Definitive Survey* (Chicago, IL: University of Chicago Press, 1994).
> 91 ."Orgasmic Dysfunction," *Medline Plus Medical Encyclopedia*, September 2002, accessed September 2012, http://www.nlm.nih.gov/medlineplus/ency/article/001953.htm.

More statistics on frequency of orgasm:

…Women are either faking it or their partners are assuming they are having an orgasm when they are not. About 85 percent of men report that their partner had an orgasm in their most recent sexual encounter. This compares to the 64 percent of women who report having had an orgasm in their most recent sexual encounter. (This difference is too large to be accounted for by some of the men having had male partners in their most recent encounter.)[92]

…Seventy-five percent of men and 29 percent of women "always" have orgasms with their partner.[93]

…Between 10 and 15 percent of women have *never had an orgasm*, and only 35 percent of women have ever had a vaginal orgasm.[94]

…Between 50 and 75 percent of women need clitoral stimulation and cannot have an orgasm through intercourse alone.[95]

…Women are more likely to orgasm when they engage in a variety of sex acts and when oral sex or vaginal intercourse is included. Men are more likely to orgasm when sex includes vaginal intercourse.[96]

…Women get better with age…better at their ability to orgasm, that is! Among those aged eighteen to fifty-nine, greater age for women is associated with a higher likelihood of their own orgasm (for men it is associated with a lower likelihood).[97]

… Women are much more likely to be "nearly always" or "always" orgasmic when alone than with a partner.[98]

…Many women express that their most satisfying sexual experiences entail being connected to someone, rather than solely basing satisfaction on orgasm.[99]

---

[92] Center for Sexual Health Promotion Indiana University, "Special Issue: Findings from the National Survey of Sexual Health and Behavior (NSSHB)," *Journal of Sexual Medicine*, 7, supp. 5 (2010): 243-373..

[93] Laumann, Gagnon, Michael, and Michaels, "The Social Organization of Sexuality: Sexual Practices in the United States."

[94] Birch, Robert W. and Cynthia L. Ruberg, *Pathways to Pleasure: A Woman's Guide to Orgasm* (Howard, OH: Pec Publishing, 2000).

[95] Cooper, Al, "Understanding the Female Orgasm," *SciForums*, July 2003, accessed January 11, 2013, http://www.sciforums.com/showthread.php?26925-Understanding-the-female-orgasm.

[96] NSSHB, 2010. Available at http://www.iub.edu/~kinsey/resources/FAQ.html#nsshb.

[97] Ibid.

[98] Davis, C.M., et al., "Characteristics of Vibrator Use Among Women."

[99] Bridges, S.K., S.H. Lease, and C.R. Ellison, C.R., "Predicting Sexual Satisfaction in Women: Implications for Counselor Education and Training," *Journal of Counseling & Development*, vol.

...Twenty-five percent of men and 14 percent of women reported that simultaneous orgasm is a must.[100]

...Ten percent of men and 18 percent of women reported a preference for oral sex to achieve orgasm.[101]

LL: Wow. That is a lot of fodder for discussion. I don't even know where to start. I think the one that surprised me the most is that twenty-five percent of men and fourteen percent of women reported that simultaneous orgasm is a must. I used to be able to do that *occasionally,* but now it *rarely* happens. That must take a lot of practice and concentration.

CG: I think an important question to ask is this—is it important to have an orgasm? I don't think it is important to have an orgasm with sex, but I do think it is important to be able to have an orgasm with your partner. It doesn't matter how you reach orgasm with your partner—whether with your partner's hand or your hand, mouth, penetration, vibrator, penis, or even touching other parts of the body. And it is ok to have an orgasm before your partner or after your partner. And it is ok to help yourself along when you are with a partner—whether with your own hand or fantasy, or verbal or nonverbal communication.

Communication between partners is essential for a relationship and for sexuality. Communication can be in different methods—verbal, nonverbal, tactile, but much of sexuality and orgasm is about the two persons communicating. It is often difficult for orgasm to happen without communication, trust, and a willingness to let yourself be vulnerable.

But back to all of that research. Now, it is important to note that although these are all good studies from respectable sex researchers and sexologists or sex therapists, this is not an exact science. To women who orgasm sometimes or frequently or never but are HAPPY and SATISFIED, I say just skip the rest of this chapter. Why try to fix something that is not broken? A majority of women don't have the need to have an orgasm all the time or even more than they do.

If a woman is *dissatisfied*—and a lot of the patients I see are, then that is a different story, and there are absolutely ways to work on this. I think we need to dedicate the rest of the chapter to this.

82, 2 (2004): 158-166.
100 Janus, S. and C. Janus, *The Janus Report on Sexual Behavior* (New York: John Wiley & Sons, 1993).
101 Ibid.

If you are dissatisfied with your ability to orgasm, not only are you not alone, but this is so common. Most women need to have direct clitoral stimulation to experience orgasms. But think about it—if a woman is heterosexual, and she mostly has vaginal intercourse, her partner's penis does not stimulate her clitoris much when it goes in and out of her vagina. He can use his hands to do this, and some women like this. But vaginal penetration alone does not provide the kind of stimulation that is necessary for many women to reach an orgasm.

Women should consider opting more for oral sex if both partners like it. As we noted previously, almost one in five prefer oral sex to achieve orgasm.

Also, some women prefer lengthened lovemaking experiences, but some do not. And taking more time is helpful for achieving orgasm—up to a certain point—but many women will not achieve orgasm unless all the stars are aligned, so even if a woman's partner continues for hours, it won't necessarily result in an orgasm.

There is a great book that I recommend to my patients called *The Elusive Orgasm*[102] by Vivienne Cass, PhD. It breaks down some of the orgasm difficulties into five types. There's ordinary "garden-variety" orgasm difficulty, women who have never had an orgasm, women who rarely have an orgasm, women who used to be able to orgasm, and women who can orgasm at some times, but not others. Then the book discusses twenty-five potential causes for the different types of difficulties, and what women can do about them.

Women's orgasms are a very complex blend of many different physical and psychological variables. Most women (but not all) have to be comfortable and happy with their partner, themselves, and the situation. Is the baby crying? Is this relationship right for me? Do I have time to have sex AND get the groceries? Does he love me? Is she too attached to me?

LL: You see what I mean about how our brains are our biggest sex organs?

CG: And it is so true. If we are feeling anxious, upset, tired, or any one of a hundred other emotions, we may not be able to have an orgasm. Men on average have a much easier time than women do. But they also often have to be in the mood or feel like the situation is right—though not as much as women do.

And as we mentioned before, men and women often reach orgasm very differently. If you are in a heterosexual relationship, and if you touch a man's penis, squeeze his shaft with the right amount of pressure, make sure to go over his

---

102 Vivienne Cass, *The Elusive Orgasm: A Woman's Guide to Why She Can't and How She Can Orgasm*, (New York: Marlowe & Co., 2007).

glans, and add some lubrication into the mix—either saliva or cream or, of course, vaginal lubrication if you are having intercourse—then all he usually needs is friction to have an orgasm. Now this may be simplifying things. This is true for many men and especially for younger men. As men get older it is increasingly more difficult to get an erection for many men, though not all.

Sexual response for women, on average, is more complex. If you plotted orgasms on a graph, a man's orgasm would on average look like one straight line going up at an angle while a woman's orgasm is more like a set of stairs. A woman usually needs some stimulation, and then she regroups, and then a bit more stimulation (maybe not the same kind), and then she regroups, and then after a few more steps she is sort of pushed over the edge and has an orgasm.

Something else that plays into whether or not a woman can have an orgasm is the messages she received about sex when she was growing up. I had a patient who had years and years and layers and layers of negative messages when it came to sex. Her mother told her that sex was dirty and that her body—especially her vagina and breasts—need to be covered up at all times. She was chided if she even tried to show her figure. As she got older, her father called her a slut if she even uttered a boy's name in the house. She was not allowed to date nor have any kind of relationships with any males. Her parents had irrational fears of her having sex at an early age, so they did not allow her to show any of her femininity.

LL: That is terrible.

CG: And it did a lot to her psyche. She's not alone—there are millions of women who have stories like that. This one patient of mine went through years of therapy before she even got to me. She had been married and divorced three times. She didn't have any children of her own. And she was just miserable. I think she got to be fifty and had a scare with lung cancer when she decided she didn't want to die without ever experiencing an orgasm. So the therapist she had been seeing for the previous eight years sent her to me. I happen to know that this therapist had tried to send her to me in the past, but she had not been open to it. I think this cancer scare and maybe just getting older and relaxing a bit…I think fifty is this magic number where many women throw caution to the wind and say, "Screw it! I'm not gonna suffer/feel self-conscious/worry/care/and so on ANY more." So she came to me and we worked on her getting an orgasm, and guess what—she did it!

LL: Wow—when was that, and how is she doing now?

CG: That was a few years ago. To tell you the truth, I don't know how she is doing now. Lots of patients I keep in touch with and see from time to time. We have a very trusting and intimate relationship while they are in my care, and they are telling me their deepest and darkest secrets during the hour or so I see them each week for months on end. But this one woman was an anomaly. She learned to orgasm one minute and she was gone the next! And I was so happy for her. So thrilled. No one should have to suffer for so long.

LL: Suffer by not having an orgasm?

CG: Well, no, that is not what I meant—suffer with those negative thoughts that brought her all that negative energy about her sexuality over the years. She was a good person, a smart, sweet person. And those negative messages growing up really did a doozy on her.

LL: Is there something we can say here for our readers who might have had a similar, or even not so similar, experience—but they are still carrying those negative feelings with them? Can we help them feel better? You know that I'm a counselor and my heart goes out to anyone who is suffering in any way.

CG: I think that a lot of it just comes down to a woman saying to herself "enough is enough" and then consciously deciding to get the negative messages out of her brain and out of her life. This is not so easy. Many women read self-help books and other women speak with trusted friends and counselors. A lot of it also comes down to practice—first being able to recognize any negative messages you send yourself and then being able to replace the negative messages with positive ones.

And so much of it comes down to this. As we've already said many times, orgasms and sex in general are just good for you. And some women, because of their psychological feelings about sex or their resistance to something that feels good, are not able to benefit from sex and orgasms because their brains are getting in their way. This is really the bottom line of why we want women to feel comfortable with their vaginas and sex—it is healthy.

LL: But do you need to have an orgasm to get all of the health benefits that were listed in the chapter on Sexuality and Intimacy?

CG: Thank goodness, no—after all, women have a longer life expectancy than men, yet they have significantly fewer orgasms! The health benefits are not dependent on having an orgasm, or even having sexual intercourse or penetration. "Orgasm is an *experience*, not a goal…Many people have satisfying sexual experiences without orgasm."[103] The bottom line is feeling good, both physically and emotionally. That is what I tell my patients, and that is really what it comes down to.

This is something I recommend to women who have never or rarely had an orgasm:

> ### *Never Had an Orgasm? Try this!*
>
> First, it is important to note that it is OK if you have never had an orgasm or if you rarely have orgasms. If you put too much pressure on yourself to have an orgasm, it can backfire. So first and foremost, tell yourself that this is going to be fun, and if it happens, it happens, but not to worry if it does not!
>
> Next sit back, relax, and try this:
>
> (1) Decide if you are going to try this by yourself or with a partner—either way is great.
>
> (2) Be sure you have privacy—no kids knocking on doors, no neighbors calling, turn off your cell phone, and so on.
>
> (3) First try a good fantasy. What turns you on? You don't know? Search the web—or go to a bookstore—or order some porn and watch it. Or read the fantasy chapter again and check out pages one hundred fifty-five through one hundred fifty-seven for good ideas for fantasies. See which one makes you feel aroused—and by aroused I mean that feeling at the bottom of your stomach and the top of your vagina—that good feeling that sort of takes you off guard.
>
> (4) Concentrate on your fantasy. Imagine yourself *in* your fantasy. If you are doing this with a partner, decide whether you are going to share the fantasy or whether it is going to remain in your head.
>
> (5) When you start to feel aroused—or even if you do not yet—then stroke your body in the way that it likes to be touched. Touch your breasts, your nipples, your inner thighs.

---

[103] Barry R. Komisaruk, Beverly Whipple, Sara Nesserzadeh, and Carlos Beyer-Flores, *The Orgasm Answer Guide* (Baltimore, MD: Johns Hopkins University Press, 2009), 110.

(6) Put your fingers near your clitoris. Don't put them directly on your clitoris because that may hurt or irritate. Remember, your clitoris is much more than the small part that shows itself to the outside world — it is also connected to the clitoral shaft, and then the crura, or legs of the clitoris. The crura are two to three inches long and lie under the inner lips, along the pelvic bones, so if you press down on your mons pubis and your vulva, your clitoris is still getting much of the stimulation.

(7) Enjoy your body for a while. Enjoy the feelings. Enjoy your fantasy. Or drop your fantasy and just focus on the physical touch and response.

(8) As you start to feel more aroused, change the speed of your pressing or touching or your fingers stimulating your clitoris. If speeding up causes you to be more aroused, then continue in this way.

(9) If you notice a decrease in arousal, this is normal. Women usually experience increases and decreases in arousal before reaching an orgasm.

(10) Continue this as if you are climbing the steps of a stairway. Appreciate all the feelings. Enjoy the responses your body makes. Enjoy the lubrication and any liquid that comes out of your vagina. Relish the swelling that you feel in your vagina and entire area. These thoughts may feel good or normal or new or surprising. But they are completely appropriate and they should not feel shameful. If your body wants to moan or make noise, allow it to.

(11) Continue this until you feel a crescendo building up. Revel in the feelings. Allow yourself to be carried up and over the top of the staircase and tumble down the other side. Delight in the rhythmic contractions and the pulsating feelings. If it feels right, then continue stimulating your clitoris to deepen the orgasm. If not, then enjoy the sense of release and relief…how your body feels when the hormones rush in to make you feel happy, sleepy, excited, or satisfied.

Suggested Resources:

Barbach, Lonnie Garfield, *For Yourself: The Fulfillment of Female Sexuality* (New York: Signet, 2001).

Betty Dodson with Carlin Ross website and blog: Better Orgasms, Better World. http://dodsonandross.com/.

Cass, Vivienne, *The Elusive Orgasm: A Woman's Guide to Why She Can't and How She Can Orgasm* (New York: Marlowe & Co., 2007).

Heiman, Julia and Joseph LoPiccolo, *Becoming Orgasmic: A Sexual and Personal Growth Program for Women* (New York: Fireside, 1987).

Komisaruk, Barry R., Beverly Whipple, Sara Nesserzadeh, and Carlos Beyer-Flores, *The Orgasm Answer Guide* (Baltimore, MD: Johns Hopkins University Press, 2009).

Lloyd, Elisabeth, *The Case of the Female Orgasm: Bias in the Science of Evolution* (Boston, MA: Harvard University Press, 2006).

CHAPTER 16

Sex!

LL: Out of curiosity I just did a Google search for the word *sex* and guess how many items came up?

CG: I have no idea. A million?

LL: One billion, seven hundred and seventy million! I knew that sex was important, but wow—I wonder if it is the most searched term on the Internet.

So sex is good for us, and it overlaps a great deal with intimacy. But what about just SEX—sex for sex's sake?

CG: You have come to the right place. I have lots to say about this! For one thing, there are a lot of people out there having a lot of sex. Females between thirty and forty-four report an average of four male sexual partners in their lifetime.[104] And interestingly, 31 percent only had one partner and nine percent had eleven or more partners.[105] But there is a good chance that these figures are low because they are self-reported. As we know, research is not an exact science, and women are scared of "slut-shaming," so they may change their "numbers" to seem more "appropriate."

LL: It is amazing that in this day and age women are still worried about this. I am not being critical, just amazed. I went with a group of eight women to a getaway weekend at a friend's lake house a few years ago, and we had the discussion about "numbers" — you know, numbers of sexual partners we have ever had. At first we were tentative talking about it. We were all married, all had kids, and we were all professionals, although some of us were not working at the time. I remember the first person said "three" and then someone else said "four." One said she had only been with her husband. I thought to myself, "Should I admit how many men I have slept with?" I mean, I wasn't ashamed, and I didn't have any regrets. But my number was way different from what everyone else was saying. Another woman said "three" — and then I had a quick "be authentic" reminder (something I remind myself of often when I feel like I can't be myself for some reason because I *know* it is always best to be myself and that the more I practice being my *true* self…the more I keep my focus on my own internal scorecard and don't focus on what others think, the better off I am). So I said, "Sixteen." One of my close friends said, "Six-teen?" in amazement. I don't think she was being judgmental — maybe just surprised. I have no problem with this number at all. I didn't have sex until I was twenty, but I met my husband, Marc, when I was thirty and had one false-start marriage and lots of boyfriends in between. In fact, if I had known then what I know now, I would have slept with more men, and I would have experimented more. I was always very cautious and always used protection. Well, except once…and then I couldn't sleep for three days, worrying I would get a sexually transmitted infection. I called the guy I had slept with and gushed about how

---

104 Mosher, Chandra, and Jones, "Sexual Behavior and Selected Health Measures: Men and Women 15–44 Years of Age, United States, 2002." Men report more partners — men aged thirty to forty-four report an average of six to eight female sexual partners in their lifetime.

105 Three percent of women have had zero sexual partners since the age of 18, 31 percent have had one partner, 36 percent have had two to four partners, 20 percent have had five to ten partners, 6 percent have had eleven to twenty partners, and 3 percent have had twenty-one or more partners. Fifty-six percent of American men and 30 percent of American women have had five or more sex partners in their lifetime (Laumann, Gagnon, Michael, and Michaels, 1994).

worried I was, and he said he had been worried, too. Luckily, we both tested negative, and I only beat myself up for a few years over that mistake.

CG: Wow. I definitely grew up in a different generation—the one right in between the sexual revolution, where everyone was having sex with everyone else, and your generation. Most women I know met their husbands in high school or college and as far as I know have never had sex with anyone else. I think the choice a woman makes is very personal and individual. I know many couples with excellent sex lives who have only had one partner as well as men and women who have had many partners. Excellent sexuality is about understanding your body and communicating with your partner, trusting, being vulnerable, all in a healthy, loving environment.

As a medical professional I do worry about the idea of sanctioning the idea that it is OK to have a lot of sexual partners. Because in the same breath, I feel the need to say that women must be safe and use protection—condoms or dental dams to be specific. And this is just a minimum—there are still diseases women can get from being intimate in other ways, like kissing!

So were you glad you admitted your number to your friends?

LL: I hate to even think of it as *admitting* it because I don't think of it as a bad thing. After I said that, another friend—a bit more quietly—said, "My number is probably closer to yours because of my wild teenage and college days."

The truth is, it really doesn't matter what our numbers are. If we are being true to ourselves—having sex because *we* want to or *not* having sex because we *don't* want to—then that is really what is most important.

Plus, look at the double standard in our society. There are some men who try to sleep with as many women as they can. But our culture just accepts this as normal—a boys-will-be-boys mentality. Cultures all around the world accept this. I don't think it is fair to have this double standard.

> Join the Revolution! *Do Not Feel One Iota of Embarrassment for the Number of Sexual Partners You Have Had—or Have Not Had*
>
> So you are a sexual person? So you slept around? So what? Women in our culture—in most cultures really—have been socialized to NOT sleep around...but are men socialized to not sleep around? No. This is because we still have a patriarchal mindset. It *used to* be that women

> did not have the right to own property or inherit money or vote, so we had to depend on a husband or father or brother or son. Now we have rights, but we are still quick to feel like we can't do what men can do. Men (on average) are so much more comfortable with their sexuality. Why aren't we?
>
> It is now acceptable in most cultures to have sex before marriage, but so many women still feel the societal pressure to *not have too much* sex. Why? Why not challenge these cultural norms? As long as you are not hurting yourself or anyone else, and of course are fully protected, then why should it matter?
>
> So you have only been with one person? Or you have never been with anyone? Or you are not currently with someone? So what? Are you comfortable with this? If so, then great. If not, then it is time to make changes. But do what *you* want, not what society says you should want.

CG: Something else notable is that women are starting to have sex much earlier than we used to—probably because in the United States and most Western countries, the stigma of sex-before-marriage is mostly gone in most subcultures. Although the average age for women to start having sex is 17.4,[106] about one quarter of women start having sex by age fifteen.

LL: I have been amazed by how many of my thirteen- and fourteen-year-old students are sexually active. And since I have been working with them since sixth grade, and now they are in eighth grade, I hear increasingly more stories from more students.

CG: One other thing to consider is that sex has a very different level of importance in each of our lives, and also for each of us over time. If you ask a hundred women how important sex is in their lives, you will hear answers ranging from "It's the be-all and end-all" to "I'm neutral about sex" to "Sex? What's that?"

And as you mentioned, there is a ton of information out there on sex. We could spend weeks talking about this topic. There is so much information about sex and so many topics that we could not possibly include them all in this book, so I will focus on two topics and then list some good go-to reference books. First, variations of sex—anal, oral, lesbian, and so on. Second, sex over time. I will

---

[106] *Sexual and Reproductive Health: Women and Men*, (New York: Alan Guttmacher Institute, 2002), accessed July 2012, http://www.guttmacher.org/pubs/fb_10-02.html.

also include go-to information about contraception and sexually transmitted infections as well.

Different Kinds of Sex

CG: A vast majority of women report that sex is an important part of their lives. Not all women do. Women can fall anywhere on the scale from "I couldn't live without it" to "I can take it or leave it!" and all attitudes are completely "normal." But considering that a majority of women do think it is important, it is interesting to ask what they mean when they say or hear the word *sex*.

When people report "having sex," they are not necessarily describing what any one reader thinks about as her normal sex life. There is enormous variability in the sexual repertoires of U.S. adults, with more than forty combinations of sexual activity described as having taken place at various adults' most recent sexual encounters.[107]

The National Survey of Sexual Health and Behavior (NSSHB) at the Kinsey Institute did a comprehensive study of the percentage of Americans performing certain sexual behaviors in the past year, and the results were fascinating. Here are results for women ages twenty-five and older. To find results for younger women or for men, readers can also go to the website http://www.nationalsexstudy.indiana.edu/.

Percentage of Americans Performing Certain Sexual Behaviors in the Past Year (N=5865)[108]

Sexual Behaviors	Women 25–29	Women 30–39	Women 40–49	Women 50–59	Women 60–69	Women 70+
Masturbated Alone	72%	63%	65%	54%	47%	33%
Masturbated with Partner	48%	43%	35%	18%	13%	5%
Received Oral from Women	3%	5%	2%	1%	1%	2%
Received Oral from Men	72%	59%	52%	34%	25%	8%

---

107 NSSHB, 2010.
108 NSSHB, 2010.

Gave Oral to Women	3%	4%	3%	1%	1%	2%
Gave Oral to Men	76%	59%	53%	36%	23%	7%
Vaginal Intercourse	87%	74%	70%	51%	42%	22%
Received Penis in Anus	21%	22%	12%	6%	4%	1%

CG: Earlier you defined *sex*[109] as either oral sex (when one partner's mouth comes into contact with the other partner's genitals), anal sex (in which a penis goes into the partner's anus), masturbation (touching or rubbing your own genitals), or vaginal intercourse (penis in vagina if you are heterosexual, or if you are a lesbian then either "tribbing"[110] or fingers or anything else in each other's vaginas).

We already spoke at length about masturbation, so let's talk about the others.

Oral Sex

LL: It's pretty much a given that most men like receiving oral sex, right? Not to stereotype...I mean, it is the subject of so many jokes, and it is a popular theme in mainstream media. But what about women? Do you think that women love receiving oral sex as much as men do? I mean I know that I for one do not. But I know that everyone is very different...

CG: It is a lot easier to find data on how many women *engage* in oral sex than it is to find data on how many women *like* it, but if I had to guess based on what I have read and heard, more women like it than dislike it. It is safe to say that many women do like getting oral sex, many do not, and many are indifferent.

I'm sure it doesn't surprise you to hear that many women feel very self-conscious about their vaginas and do not want their partners looking at or licking them.

---

[109] A recent study at the Kinsey Institute found that nearly 45 percent of participants considered manual-genital stimulation—in slang terms, a "hand job"—as "having sex." Seventy-one percent considered oral sex to be sex, 80.8 percent for anal-genital intercourse.
[110] Tribadism (or tribbing) is a form of nonpenetrative sex in which a woman rubs her vulva against her partner's body for sexual stimulation. More information on lesbian sex is in the chapter on sexual orientation.

In my practice, I have worked with women whose partners wanted to perform oral sex, but they did not want them to. In most cases, once a woman becomes more comfortable with her vagina, then she can learn to accept and even love oral sex. But other women do not ever learn to like it. And that is fine—to each her own.

One advantage of oral sex is that it enables women to orgasm more easily in many cases (though not all) because it provides direct stimulation to the clitoris. Plus, the tongue is very sensitive and saliva provides extra lubrication. The amount of pressure is different than fingers or a hand, and it seems to get better results orgasmically speaking.

As for the data on frequency:

…Half or more of women ages eighteen to thirty-nine reported giving or receiving oral sex in the past ninety days.[111]

…Receptive oral sex is reported by more than half of women between the ages of eighteen and sixty-nine who are in a cohabitating relationship. It was also reported by more than half of women cohabitating between ages eighteen and forty-nine, and more than half of married women ages thirty to thirty-nine.[112]

…A similar pattern was found for women performing oral sex.[113]

Anal Sex

LL: OK, I have to admit that I have a friend who LOVES anal sex and cannot get enough of it, but I have never tried it, nor do I have any desire to try it.

CG: Some women try it and like it, others do not, and still others can't even think about anal sex without cringing. Studies show that more and more women are trying it and liking it. In fact, the National Sex Survey reported anal sex as way up from previous surveys in previous years. I read a series of articles in *Slate* a couple of years ago about this. A writer for *Slate*, William Saletan, wrote the following in his article "The Ass Man Cometh: Experimentation, Orgasms, and the Rise of Anal Sex."

> "Here's the big story. In 1992, 16 percent of women aged 18–24 said they'd tried anal sex. Now 20 percent of women aged 18–19 say they've done it, and by ages 20–24, the number is 40 percent. In 1992, the highest percentage

---

111 NSSHB, 2010.
112 Ibid.
113 Ibid.

of women in any age group who admitted to anal sex was 33. In 2002, it was 35. Now it's 46.

The last time I looked at the anal sex data, I figured that most women who reported having done it meant they'd tried it just once. I was wrong. If you push these women beyond the "have you ever" question, the numbers stay surprisingly high, and they're getting higher. In 1992, the percentage of women in their 20s and 30s who said they'd had anal sex in the past year was around 10 percent. Now that number has doubled to more than 20 percent, and one-third of these women say they've done it in the last month."[114]

LL: Fascinating. I wonder why the numbers are up so much? Again, it is so hard for me to even imagine. But maybe that is just a mental block on my part.

CG: It probably is. There are so many women who just love anal sex. Many love it more than vaginal and oral sex.

Some women orgasm more easily having anal sex. It frees up their partner's hands to touch their breasts or vagina. Other women have more intense orgasms with anal sex—there is a connection between the sphincter muscles and the whole region.

I think other women enjoy the "adventure" of anal sex. Perhaps if they have not had anal sex, they see it as being very radical, and when they get to a point in their lives where they want to try something new—and often it is women who are within a relationship—this is one thing that is just easy to try. It is different, almost dangerous, and daring.

Some of my patients use a butt plug before having anal sex, and some lesbians use one in lieu of a penis or vibrator.

LL: Butt plug?

CG: It's a sex toy that is designed to fit in your anus and rectum for sexual pleasure. It sort of looks like a shortened vibrator, but it flares out so the whole thing can't get stuck and disappear into the depths of your bowel. (Unlike a vagina, where objects can only travel up so far before hitting a dead end at the cervix, the bowels are long, and in the heat of the moment it is easy for an object to get stuck up there.)

---

114 William Saletan, "The Ass Man Cometh: Experimentation, Orgasms, and the Rise of Anal Sex," *Slate*, October 5, 2010, accessed September 2012, http://www.slate.com/articles/health_and_science/human_nature/2010/10/the_ass_man_cometh.html.

LL: Ouch. My husband, Marc, used to be an emergency room doctor, and he has a lot of stories about people coming in with things stuck in their butts!

CG: One other thing about butt plugs—many people cover them with a condom for easy cleaning, and also they usually need lubrication and a slow, steady insertion into the anus.

Like everything else, every woman has different tastes and different ideas about everything, sex included. And for women who may be curious about anal sex—hey, it's worth a try. But this is certainly not for everyone and women will draw their own conclusions about what is right for them.

Lesbian Sex

CG: Speaking of worth a try, did you know that women who have sex with other women have significantly more orgasms than women who have sex with men?[115]

Any time any two adults are together having a sexual experience, they may engage in oral sex, anal sex, or vaginal sex, and when two women are together it is no different. The main thing that is missing is a natural, biological penis. But there are plenty of options that mimic the penetration by a penis.

LL: OK, don't laugh, but I need a little help here. I know tons of lesbians—in fact, at one point I felt like the only straight female at my former school—but I never worked up the courage to actually ask my friends about the details of lesbian sex. And I have always been curious.

CG: You've got to get out more and explore. Over a quarter of women report being aroused by another woman[116] and one in five[117] report having had some kind of physical interaction with another woman, though the percent of women who consider themselves *lesbian* is closer to eight percent and bisexual closer to nine percent.[118]

---

115 In 1953, Alfred Kinsey's *Sexual Behavior in the Human Female* showed that, over the previous five years of sexual activity, 78 percent of women had orgasms in 60 to 100 percent of sexual encounters with other women, compared with 55 percent for heterosexual sex. Other studies have replicated the results of Kinsey's original study. Alfred C. Kinsey, Wardell B. Pomeroy, Clyde E. Martin, and Paul H. Gebhard, *Sexual Behavior in the Human Female* (Philadelphia, PA: Saunders, 1953).

116 Ibid.

117 Ibid.

118 Shere Hite, *The Hite Report: A National Study of Female Sexuality* (New York: Macmillan, 1976).

Before I explain lesbian sex, I've got to point out that it also applies to women who are bisexual or experimenting, or who dispense with sexual orientation altogether. I am just talking here about women who are having sex with other women.

LL: OK.

CG: And you may read this and think that it sounds a lot like heterosexual sex, and there is good reason for that—they are very similar!

Lesbian sex is often characterized by more full-body sexual contact instead of just a focus on genitals. Women often engage in kissing, breast and nipple stimulation and fondling, and caressing each other's arms, backs, thighs, buttocks, and bodies in general.

Women also tend to engage in oral sex that involves stimulation of the woman's vulva, clitoris, or vagina. Sometimes women also practice analingus, which is oral stimulation of the anus.

Tribbing is also common when two women want to be intimate with each other. Kathy Belge helped define tribadism in a piece on About.com. "Tribadism involves rubbing your genitals against another person's genitals or other body part. Many lesbians enjoy tribadism because they can involve their whole bodies. Also called *humping*, tribadism can involve straddling a partner's leg, pubic bone, or any other body part. Many women can orgasm just from this stimulation."[119] This may be done with one woman on top or both side by side or spooning. Really any position that two women feel comfortable with can allow for the body parts to come in contact with each other erotically.

While tribadism or tribbing is a nonpenetrative sexual act between two women, there are also many common penetrative sexual acts. Women can use their fingers to massage each other's vulva, clitoris, vagina, or anus. Women may insert their fingers into each other's vaginas and try to find and massage each other's G-spots. For deeper penetration they may use a vibrator or sex toy, though Masters and Johnson found that women rarely use dildos (vibrators) with each other.[120]

LL: So what do lesbian women do the most when they are physically intimate?

---

119 Kathy Belge, "What Is Tribadism," *About.com*, n.d., accessed July 1, 2012, http://lesbian-life.about.com/od/lesbiansex/f/Tribadism.htm.
120 Jerrold S. Greenberg, Clint E. Bruess, and Sarah C. Conklin, Exploring the Dimensions of Human Sexuality (Burlington, MA: Jones & Bartlett Learning, 2010), 884.

CG: Obviously, every woman likes something different, so you cannot generalize and say all lesbians like...or all heterosexuals like... I read this great quote from sex educator and feminist Shere Hite. She noted that one of her female research subjects had written "Sex with a woman includes: touching, kissing, smiling, looking serious, embracing, talking, digital intercourse, caressing, looking, cunnilingus, undressing, remembering later, making sounds, sometimes gently biting, sometimes crying, and breathing and sighing together."[121]

LL: It does sound like she could also be talking about heterosexual sex.

CG: I read about an interesting study in 1987. It was a nonscientific study conducted among more than a hundred members of a lesbian social organization in Colorado. When asked what techniques they used in their last ten sexual encounters, one hundred percent reported kissing, sucking on breasts, and manual stimulation of the clitoris; more than ninety percent reported French kissing, oral sex, and fingers inserted into the vagina; and eighty percent reported tribadism.[122]

Vaginal Intercourse

CG: When most heterosexual people say "sex" they mean intercourse — penetration of a woman's vagina with a man's penis (PIV sex, aka penis-in-vagina). In fact, the majority of women age eighteen to forty-nine report vaginal intercourse in the past ninety days.[123]

While vaginal intercourse is still the most common sexual behavior reported by adults, many sexual events do not involve intercourse and include only partnered masturbation or oral sex.[124]

LL: Perhaps with the increase of anal sex and the increase of women liking oral sex that vaginal sex will decrease over time. I mean, if women get orgasms more easily from other kinds of sex, and men who are older can't hold an erection as easily, doesn't it make sense that the tide will turn?

CG: I don't think I would go as far as to say the tide will turn...I do think that vaginal sex will always be most popular and enjoyed — but I do agree that more and more people will be expanding their sexual repertoire, especially as

---

[121] Shere Hite, "Lesbianism: Women's Sexual Expression Together," *Hite-Research*, October 17, 2008, accessed July 1, 2012.
[122] Janell L. Carroll, *Sexuality Now: Embracing Diversity* (Belmont, CA: Wadsworth, Cengage Learning), 629.
[123] NSSHB, 2010.
[124] NSSHB, 2010.

different kinds of sex get more air time and are more prevalent in the mainstream media. Just as we talked about earlier, sexuality is innate, but the kinds of sex had in different cultures vary just like kinds of food. The "tastes" we grow up with tend to stick with us. Just as you may not have seen or heard about anal sex when you were in your more impressionable years, and so now you think you have a mental block, kids today are hearing about it more and seeing it more and so will consider it to be more natural. Almost certainly, the survey numbers will follow.

But it is true that in older couples, PIV sex is not practiced as much as among younger folks. Partly this is because of the erection issues that men face as they get older, and partly this is because, as we spoke about in Your Vagina Over Time, there is not as much vaginal lubrication after menopause and vaginal sex is not as easy as it once was.

Speaking of that, how about moving on to Sex Over Time?

Sex Over Time

CG: I would not be telling you something new if I told you that *on average* single people in their twenties have higher sex drives than, say, married people in their fifties.

LL: Ha! How about married people in their forties? Or thirties? Or how about partnered people at any age after the first year or two or three of being partnered?

CG: Exactly! There is tons of information all over, and most of us can just look at our own lives for a reminder of this.

But there are a few things worth noting. Just as you spoke about in the earlier chapter Your Vagina Over Time, sexual intercourse is more difficult for vaginas during perimenopause and menopause. Women's sex drives are often diminished thanks to the changes in hormones. Often our vaginas get dry, thanks again to our hormones, and vaginal intercourse is not as easy. And, as we mentioned earlier, men are having their own aging issues. But we must go on! Most of us like sex, and most of us agree that it is important to a relationship. And the health benefits are still there—don't forget that huge list of health benefits for being physically intimate with someone.

It is easy at this point for women to avoid having sex and for partnerships to get less physical, but I think devoting extra work and attention to the issue ends up paying off and making women happier in the long run.

LL: So what should women do?

CG: Like women everywhere, they need to work with the changes. If your vagina is less lubricated, but you still desire vaginal intercourse, invest in some lubricants such as Slippery Stuff (brand name) and use it for added lubrication. Also re-assess what works for you sexually, or perhaps look at your relationship. If your sex drive is down, speak with your doctor about hormone replacement therapy or bioidentical hormones. I know that studies have scared away some women, but if your lifestyle is seriously being affected by your lack of sex drive and your postmenopausal mood changes, then it is absolutely something to look into. There is enough controversy over this that it warrants reading up on it and getting different medical opinions. Go to your doctor, and if you don't like her opinion, get a second or third opinion.

By the way, there are many women who report an *increased* sex drive after menopause. Sometimes this is because they don't have to worry about pregnancy, sometimes it is because their children are older or out of the house, and sometimes different people's hormones just work in different ways. These women should appreciate this because it is not the case for everyone.

Women's Day magazine printed a great article by Sarah Jio titled "Sex by the Numbers." Check out this fascinating information:[125]

When it comes to sex, there are a million different numbers—from the average length of time it lasts to the number of calories a romp in the sack burns. We compiled the most interesting statistics on the topic, and ran them by our experts to see what they really mean for you.

84: Percentage of women who say they have sex to get their man to help out around the house.

200: Number of calories the average person burns during thirty minutes of sexual intercourse.

20: Percentage of Americans who have had sex with a coworker.

2: The number of minutes before ejaculation that qualifies as premature.

---

125 Sarah Jio, "Sex by the Numbers," *Woman's Day*, accessed January 11, 2013, http://www.womansday.com/sex-relationships/sex-tips/sex-by-the-numbers-103274.

> **25:** Percentage of Americans who are living with an incurable STI.
>
> **12:** Percentage of married people who sleep alone.
>
> **20:** Number of minutes the average couple spends on foreplay.
>
> **103:** Number of times per year that the average person has sex.
>
> **48:** Percentage of women who say they have faked an orgasm at least once in their life.
>
> **48:** Percentage of Americans who report being satisfied with their sex life.

Sexually Transmitted Infections

We would be remiss to have so much talk about sex and nothing about sexually transmitted infections (STI). By the way, this is the new term—STDs or sexually transmitted diseases is no longer the term being used for this. It is now STIs. One in four women has some kind of STI. Please see appendix 3 for a list of infections, symptoms, and more.

Suggested Resources:

Carnal Knowledge blog, with Dr. Jannell Carroll. http://www.drjanellcarroll.com/wordpress/.

Dr. Carroll is a professor, sex educator, and prolific blogger.

Hooper, Anne and Daphne Razazan, *Great Sex Games* (New York: DK Books, 2000).

Hutcherson, Hilda, *What Your Mother Never Told You About Sex* (New York: Perigee, 2003).

Johannides, Paul. *The Guide to Getting It On: A New and Mostly Wonderful Book About Sex for Adults of All Ages* (Saline, MI: Goofy Foot Press, 2012).

Kerner, Ian, *She Comes First: The Thinking Man's Guide to Pleasuring a Woman* (New York: William Morrow, 2010).

> The Kinsey Institute was founded by Dr. Alfred Kinsey in 1947. Their mission is to advance
>
> health and knowledge worldwide through research. Visit their website at http://www.kinseyinstitute.org/research/. They also have a fabulous, informative, and user-friendly blog—http://kinseyconfidential.org/.
>
> The National Survey of Sexual Health and Behavior (NSSHB) is an amazing and comprehensive survey of sexual attitudes and behaviors of Americans. The study was conducted by researchers from the Center for Sexual Health Promotion located at Indiana University School of Public Health-Bloomington. Other researchers who participated were from the Kinsey Institute and the Indiana University School of Medicine. For more information, see Center for Sexual Health Promotion Indiana University, "Special Issue: Findings from the National Survey of Sexual Health and Behavior (NSSHB)," *JSM*. vol. 7, supp. 5 (2010): 243-373 or visit http://www.nationalsexstudy.indiana.edu/.

Passionista: The Empowered Woman's Guide to Pleasuring a Man, (New York: William Morrow, 2008).

Love, Paticia and Jo Robinson, *Hot Monogamy: Essential Steps to More Passionate, Intimate Lovemaking* (Charleston, SC: CreateSpace, 2012).

Schnarch, David, *Passionate Marriage: Keeping Love and Intimacy Alive in Committed Relationships* (New York: W.W. Norton, 2009).

Taormino, Tristan, *The Ultimate Guide to Anal Sex for Women* (San Francisco, CA: Cleis Press, 2006).

Vennig, Rachel, Claire Cavanah and Jessica Vitkus, *Morgasam: Babeland's Guide to Mind-Blowing Sex* (New York: Avery, 2010).

PART III

VAGINA—THE SPIRIT AND SOUL

17. Childbirth and Motherhood

18. Sexual Orientation

19. Gender Identity

20. What Is Going On With Our Sisters Worldwide

21. Comfort for the Soul: Taking Care of Your Vagina *and* Yourself

22. The Word on the Word and the Final Word

PART III

VAGINA—THE SPIRIT AND SOUL

CG: Your mind really does affect your feelings about your vagina, sexuality, body and, well, everything. But do you really think that the vagina has spiritual and soulful aspects?

LL: I do. It's not that your vagina has her own spirit or soul. It's more that every woman has a spirit and a soul, and it is very interconnected with her body and her vagina.

Every woman (and man, too, of course) has her own spirit and soul, and they relate to her mind and body to make every decision she ever makes—both conscious and subconscious decisions. Whether it is the decision to have (or adopt) children or not; the inclination to be sexually attracted to men or women or both or none; the calculation about how we prioritize our time—whether we throw ourselves into our careers or our families or our friends or all of the above or none; how strongly we feel emotions, and what emotions we feel (or let ourselves feel); and the ways we process past experiences; and the ways we deal with both positive and negative ones. And because our vaginas play such a large part in many of our lives, they are affected by all of the above, in a very complex interplay between our physical bodies, our minds, and our spirits and souls.

The soul can be defined as being your "unique individual identity"—that which makes you, *you* and nobody else. You are not just your personality, but your DNA, your cells, your brain, your synapses and the way that they connect messages in your brain, your looks, your hormones, your emotions, your thoughts, your past experiences, your everything. It is so difficult—maybe impossible—to hold a whole soul in one body. It's like it is too big to be tied down to one body. Your soul encompasses your body but also goes *beyond* your physical body.

The idea of a woman's *spirit* and *soul* often overlap because they both contrast with her body, but in fact they are different entities. Thousands of philosophers, poets, and others all have different ideas of what the words *spirit* and *soul* mean.

Many women believe that every living thing has a soul—even that the universe has a soul.

And spirit can be defined as the *energy* or life force in all living things. You cannot quite put your finger on it, but you know it is there.

CG: So tell me again what the spirit and soul have to do with vaginas? This is really a very complex idea.

LL: It is. I think it is better understood by breaking it down. There are infinite ways in which soul and spirit are intertwined with being a woman. We can't possibly cover all of the ways, but let's touch on a few that are relevant to many women. Let's first talk about the idea of childbirth and being a mother and how that interconnects with a woman's spirit and soul—maybe that will better help explain the connection between a woman's vagina and her spirit and soul.

CHAPTER 17

Childbirth and Motherhood

LL: A vast majority of women in the United States (80 percent) have children.[126] But many do not. Some want children and cannot have them. Others have them and do not want them, or have a great deal of ambivalence about wanting them. Some became pregnant accidentally and did not want children, but learned to love them, and now cannot imagine their lives without children. Many are still undecided. Just as there are many different shapes and sizes of

---

[126] It's interesting to note that 20 percent of women ages forty to forty-four have not had children, and that this is double the figure from thirty years ago: http://www.nytimes.com/2008/08/19/us/19census.html?_r=1.

faces and labia, so too are there many different reasons for having or not having a child.

And even women who don't or can't have children still have to address the social expectation that "women have children." Women are frequently asked "Do you have children?" So mothering actually affects all women in some way, even if we are not all mothers.

This chapter speaks more to women who have had children — whether through adoption or birth. In this chapter, I try to explain how a woman's spirit and soul intersects with her experience with childbirth and becoming a mother.

***

LL: So what do you think about when you think about childbirth?

CG: That's easy. I think about the first-, second-, third-, and even fourth-degree tears that happen during delivery. Then I think about working with the women who have had these tears on trying to get their pelvic floors toned and the sensations back — if they lose any sensation, that is.

LL: No, no, I mean what do you think about childbirth *in general*? What about having your own babies?

CG: Hmm. Well, I'm from a different generation than you are. In my generation, we didn't really think about these things as much. We just did them. The basic expectation of women was that they would go to college, meet a man, focus on a career — or not — and then get married and have children. And we considered ourselves more progressive than the generation before us — our mothers — who mostly did not have a career, and in many cases also did not go to college.

LL: OK, so the path was sort of set, and you went down the path. What about now? Are you glad you had children?

CG: I consider myself lucky. The path that was set was one that I probably would have wanted to go on anyway had I actually actively *thought* about it. I was young when I got married and pregnant. I really loved being pregnant. And delivery was the most spectacular experience of my life.

LL: For me, I knew that I wanted to have children since I was a child. I knew it was the purpose of my life. I know you are scientific, and you may say that I was socialized to want children, or that I was genetically programmed to want babies. And you may be right. But the way I see it and feel it, is that from the bottom of my soul, I wanted to have children and wanted to raise them. It didn't matter to me whether the children were my biological children. For years I thought I was going to be infertile, so I gave a lot of thought to adoption. But in any case, I would not have considered my life complete had I not had children. For me, I think that was my soul talking.

CG: Yes, but how do you define that? How do you quantify it? How do you explain it?

LL: I don't know—just as I did?

For many women the *experience* of childbirth is a spiritual one. Many women find that their bodies work with their minds and souls from pregnancy to birth and beyond. Some women are amazed and some overwhelmed by the miracle of carrying a baby inside their bodies or even expelling the baby from their bodies. Women who adopt babies and children have also described it as spiritual—to know that you are going to be caring for and nurturing another human being. I think that all of this is spiritual, and so profound. Can't we just leave it at that, or do you need a scientific description?

CG: I guess it is hard to put your finger on such an abstract idea…

LL: Although childbirth can be a spiritual experience for many, it is not always this way—either because the mother does not see it this way or because something else gets in the way of the experience of *feeling* spiritual. I had the chance recently to speak with a friend of a friend of mine who is a retired midwife. She told me the story of when she had her first child in the 1960s. Her male OB/GYN was *old school,* and even though she wanted to be awake and part of her delivery, he gave her drugs to put her to sleep. Later he explained to her "I can't have you women getting in the way of me taking your babies!" My friend woke up in a recovery room without her baby and later learned that her baby was in the nursery, and that she would not get to see her daughter until the next day at noon. This was such a disheartening experience for her, and she described it as hurting her soul. It was as if her daughter had been ripped from her body and ripped from her soul. Luckily for her, she was reunited with her baby the next day, and they have had a loving relationship since then—for forty-plus years. When I heard her story, it felt a bit like my soul was being torn as well.

This experience led her to go into the field of nursing and become a midwife. She was able to give most women the kind of birthing experiences they wanted.

She said that she helped deliver over a thousand babies over the course of fifteen years, and I asked her to tell us a bit about her experiences.

CG: With the experiences I have had, I can safely say that the vagina is the most forgiving part of the body. And just like a woman's soul, her vagina can take an incredible amount of stretching and tearing and still bounce back to (almost) its former self.

LL: What are some of the things you have learned through your experiences?

CG: Wow. How to summarize over a thousand births? I feel so lucky to have been with so many women for such momentous times in their lives. One big theme, however, was the idea of vulnerability and empowerment. Most of the women in my generation—and I am in my sixties— felt vulnerable when going into the birthing process. They did not have much say in how their babies were delivered. Now, I am generalizing here a bit. I am sure there were some exceptions. But women back then had less control over their lives in general. Women did not have the range of choices for careers that they do now—if their husband or community even accepted working women.

Today it is much different. Women have more choices. Birthing plans, where women can research and then write down a plan for how they want their births to go, are common. They can choose to have an epidural, or pain medication, or not. Or they can change their minds midway through labor. They can choose who is in the delivery room with them. They can choose to have their baby at home or in a tub at the hospital or birthing center. Having more choices makes women feel more empowered, and thus more aligned with their values and desires.

LL: This is a more soulful way to go through this very powerful experience. But even today, some women feel like they don't have ownership over their own birth experience. Many women have a *fear* of being able to give birth without intervention, and so they hand the process over to medical professionals. And fear in general gets in the way of a woman being able to listen to her soul—her inner self that has ideas about what she wants. Sometimes when a woman experiences fear, this emotion drowns out what her soul really desires.

Every woman should be empowered to choose what kind of birth experience she wants—if she wants an epidural or pain medication, then that is what she should have. If she wants natural childbirth without any drugs, then she should have that.

> Join the Revolution! **Take charge of your birth experience!**
>
> Every woman should be able to have the kind of birth experience she wants. But before this happens, she should explore all available options. She should speak with women who have had a variety of different experiences, including natural childbirth, childbirth with drugs, C-sections, and so on. She should speak with women who are not necessarily in her circle of friends to get opinions from outside her comfort zone. She should especially speak with her doctor or midwife. If the medical professional she is working with is not on the same page as she is then she should consider interviewing other medical professionals and perhaps changing to work with someone else. And then she should choose the kind of experience she wants to have. Try looking at these books for different ideas: *The Thinking Woman's Guide to a Better Birth* by Henci Goer and *Mind Over Labor: A Breakthrough Guide to Giving Birth* by Carl Jones, Marian Thompson, and Emmett E. Miller.
>
> But just as importantly as a woman knowing what kind of birth experience she wants is knowing that it is extremely important to be flexible and to be willing to change mid-stream if that is what is needed or wanted. For example no matter how much a woman wants to have a vaginal delivery if the baby is in danger and the medical professional recommends a C-section then of course that is what should happen. Women need to work with nature *and* their medical professionals to do what is best for the baby. It is great to have Plan A, Plan B and even Plan C, and ultimately be at peace if Plan A does not work out.

LL: In all of the experiences you had with delivering babies, did you find women to be comfortable and at peace with their vaginas?

CG: The kind of women I worked with were probably already more likely to be comfortable in general than the general population. After all, I was a midwife, and the vast majority of women were still choosing to have OB/GYNs deliver their babies.

I encouraged women to look at their vaginas and cervixes to give them a better idea of their bodies and what would be happening during childbirth. I would say that about a third of women wanted to look at their open vaginas and see where their cervix was, a third definitely did not want to look anywhere down there, and a third could be persuaded.

One thing I find absolutely fascinating about childbirth is how incredibly mind-boggling our bodies are. I find it very spiritual just to think about this. The fact that a woman's body can get pregnant and carry a baby to term is a miracle. And our hormones play a fascinating role in childbirth and delivery as well. Did you know that the same hormone—oxytocin—that is the "feel-good" hormone released at the time of orgasm is also released at the time of birth? It causes the vagina to contract, it causes the uterus to contract, and when a woman breastfeeds, her oxytocin increases to help her body get back to its pre-pregnant state.

LL: I'm back to feeling like maybe we are all just a big pile of hormones!

This topic is so complex because so much feeling comes along with the territory of becoming a mother. So much joy…so much fear…some pain…and I'm not just talking about childbirth. I think there is even more pain when our hearts ache over our children—whether over something major, like our child having a serious health condition or the seemingly minor but still painful pang when you hear about your child being shunned by a friend.

It reminds me of the e-mail that always circulates sometime around Mother's Day…the one where the daughter asks the mother if she and her husband should have a baby…

CG: I love that e-mail! Would you print it below? Even though I have seen it around every Mother's Day for the past five years, it still makes me weep when I read it.

From e-mail chain mail: **Being a Mom**[127]

We are sitting at lunch one day when my daughter casually mentions that she and her husband are thinking of starting a family. "We're taking a survey," she says, half joking. "Do you think I should have a baby?"

"It will change your life," I say, carefully keeping my tone neutral. "I know," she says. "No more sleeping in on weekends and no more spontaneous vacations."

---

[127] Author unknown.

But that is not what I meant at all. I look at my daughter, trying to decide what to tell her. I want her to know what she will never learn in childbirth classes. I want to tell her that the physical wounds of childbearing will heal, but becoming a mother will leave her with an emotional wound so raw that she will forever be vulnerable. I consider warning her that she will never again read a newspaper without asking, "What if that had been MY child?"

That every plane crash, every house fire will haunt her. That when she sees pictures of starving children, she will wonder if anything could be worse than watching your child die. I look at her carefully manicured nails and stylish suit and think that no matter how sophisticated she is, becoming a mother will reduce her to the primitive level of a bear protecting her cub. That an urgent call of "Mom!" will cause her to drop a soufflé or her best crystal without a moment's hesitation.

I feel that I should warn her that no matter how many years she has invested in her career, she would be professionally derailed by motherhood. She might arrange for childcare, but one day she will be going into an important business meeting and she will think of her baby's sweet smell…and she will have to use every ounce of discipline to keep from running home, just to make sure her baby is all right.

I want my daughter to know that everyday decisions will no longer be routine. That a five-year-old boy's desire to go to the men's room rather than the women's at McDonald's will become a major dilemma. That right there, in the midst of clattering trays and screaming children, issues of independence and gender identity will be weighed against the prospect that a child molester may be lurking in that restroom.

However decisive she may be at the office, she will second-guess herself constantly as a mother. Looking at my attractive daughter, I want to assure her that eventually she will shed the pounds of pregnancy, but she will never feel the same about herself. That her life, now so important, will be of less value to her once she has a child. That she would give herself up in a moment to save her offspring, but will also begin to hope for more years, not to accomplish her own dreams, but to watch her child accomplish theirs.

> I want her to know that a cesarean scar or shiny stretch marks will become badges of honor. My daughter's relationship with her husband will change and not in the way she thinks. I wish she could understand how much more you can love a man who is careful to powder the baby or who never hesitates to play with his child. I think she should know that she would fall in love with him again for reasons she would now find very unromantic. I wish my daughter could sense the bond she will feel with women throughout history who have tried to stop war, prejudice, and drunk driving.
>
> I want to describe to my daughter the exhilaration of seeing your child learn to ride a bike. I want to capture for her the belly laugh of a baby who is touching the soft fur of a dog or cat for the first time. I want her to taste the joy that is so real it actually hurts.
>
> My daughter's quizzical look makes me realize that tears have formed in my eyes. "You'll never regret it," I finally say. Then I reach across the table, squeeze my daughter's hand and offer a silent prayer for her, and for me, and for all the mere mortal women who stumble their way into this most wonderful of callings.

CG: Yep, here come the tears.

LL: Reading that e-mail again confirms that having a child is an emotional, rational, and spiritual decision. If the decision to have a child is aligned with your soul's desire and longing, it can be a really wonderful thing. After having my first child, Max, I got a card that read "I carried you under my heart for nine months, and in it for every second of every day since". I got that card framed, and it is hung near my bed because it really does sum up so much of motherhood. Becoming a mother permanently alters you. It changes your body—even if you adopt—because your heart is now "worn on the outside of your body." It changes your mind—you cannot possibly think the same way that you did before…and it changes your soul.

CG: But even though there is so much beauty and wonder and love surrounding having a child, it is important to remember that it is not this way for everyone. The vast majority of women recovery easily from childbirth. I tend to see women who have medical conditions often caused by the trauma of childbirth. They have rips and tears, and intercourse is painful for them. Often I can fix the problems, but occasionally surgery is needed for repair. In rare occasions women's vaginas are changed by childbirth and are never quite the same.

LL: I thought they were never quite the same, period. I know mine was not.

CG: True, and I know we touched on the physical problems that can occur post childbirth back in the section on Vagina: The Body. But we didn't touch on the changes that occur to the woman's mind, spirit, and soul from having children. A good example of this is postpartum depression.

Postpartum Depression

CG: Many women get postpartum depression and have a difficult time bonding with or caring for their babies after giving birth to them. According to research from the Centers for Disease Control (CDC) between eleven and eighteen percent of women suffer from postpartum depression.[128] Even more suffer from the baby blues.

LL: Remember when Brooke Shields made this issue more public when she spoke publicly about her postpartum depression?

CG: Yes, and Tom Cruise—that jerk—said he did not believe in postpartum depression. What an idiot. When has he ever experienced female hormonal changes? I have not been able to see a movie with Tom Cruise in it since he said that.

LL: One of my best friends, Eve, had bad postpartum depression after having her first baby. It was really miserable. She felt like she should be really happy, and she was not.

I remember definitely having the postpartum *blues* after having Max. What I remember most is that every little thing would set me off—I would cry at the words of a song, and I would feel overwhelmed when trying to nurse. I felt like I wasn't "a natural" at raising a baby. And I was thirty-three years old and married when I had him. I can only imagine how overwhelmed younger women with less of a support system might feel when they have babies.

CG: If you analyze the statistics you will see that almost one million women each year in the United States alone suffers from postpartum depression.[129] If

---

[128] Centers for Disease Control, accessed January 2013, http://www.cdc.gov/reproductive-health/Depression/index.htm

[129] John W. Schmitt, "Depression During and After Pregnancy: Frequently Asked Questions," USHHS, March 3, 2009, accessed October 2012, http://www.womenshealth.gov/publications/our-publications/fact-sheet/depression-pregnancy.pdf.

you know of anyone who is weepy after giving birth or who feels overwhelmed and hopeless, then please suggest to her that she see a doctor immediately. Women sometimes feel that they are *supposed to* be ecstatic after giving birth, and then if they are not, they may feel guilty and ashamed on top of the postpartum depression. I wish I could tell them not to feel badly about this. They did not do anything to deserve it! And they should not feel badly about getting help for it. There are great books and websites that can explain in more detail what postpartum depression is, and also how to tell the difference between that and the "blues," which can just be a temporary emotion that follows the major hormonal shifts of pregnancy and childbirth. Here is one great website where the U.S. Department of Health and Human Services Office on Women's Health offers relevant information http://www.womenshealth.gov/publications/our-publications/fact-sheet/depression-pregnancy.cfm. They_as also have a hotline to call if women have questions about pregnancy, breastfeeding, depression, and other topics. The number is 1-800-994-9662.

It is EXTREMELY important for a mother to go to her doctor when in doubt—not just for her own sake, but also for the sake of her baby, who can be in danger if she does not go. Babies tend to take on the depression—or anxiety—of their mothers, and if a mother can change this, it will benefit the baby, possibly for her whole lifetime.

LL: One thing that women are often unaware of after having children is that sometimes their body is not in balance or alignment with their spirit and soul. It could be because of the trauma of childbirth or the hormonal changes or because they are trying to fit their old images of themselves into the new roles and responsibilities of being a mother. Or it can just be sheer exhaustion and sleep deprivation.

Many women feel the same kind of shame after having children as they experience with their bodies in general—the shame we spoke about earlier in the book, where women feel uncomfortable about or embarrassed about their bodies or their thoughts.

I have to admit that at the time I was having the postpartum blues, I was not really aware that I was having the blues. I mean I knew that I was crying a lot. But I think that I felt an undercurrent of shame about feeling sad. I had just given birth to a healthy baby boy, and I was "supposed" to be feeling joy, and I was not.

I felt the undercurrent of "shame" when it comes to mothering in another way as well. Being an educated woman, I knew about the importance of bonding with your baby. Bonding with your baby is one of the most important gifts you could give to him or her. It becomes the basis of all other relationships your child will have throughout his or her life. Sometimes bonding is affected by postpartum depression, and sometimes it is affected by the mother having some kind of resistance to having a new baby or babies.

When I had Max and even Kate, my second child, I still had not *let go* of the person I was before having children. My spirit and soul were torn. I knew that I *should* bond with my children, but I was so used to being an individual. I was very independent and not used to having such intense connections. My connections with my husband, parents, and friends were always very good and loving, but never intense. And all of a sudden there was this being in my life who was completely dependent on me. I was nursing, so I could not be out of reach for more than two hours because pumping just did not work for me. I was feeling swallowed up by this new role I was supposed to be good at, and it did not feel natural.

CG: Were you still working?

LL: I was working at the time for an Internet business, and I was on maternity leave for three months. But I felt flooded—overwhelmed with responsibility and angst and anxiety about being able to raise a child. Even though it is easy for me now to speak about evolving, learning, and growing, when I was actually experiencing this new experience, I felt very smothered and dazed. And this made me feel very ashamed, so I tried to hide it even more and bury it deep within me.

As a result of all this I did not feel like I could bond very well with Max. Even though I loved him and said—and I am sure I would—that I would die for him from the moment he was born. But despite knowing rationally that I would give my life for him, when it came down to my emotions I still felt so conflicted.

CG: So did you go talk to someone? How long did it last?

LL: I eventually did get counseling, but in retrospect I should have gone sooner. Which is why I am writing about this here—hoping that someone who reads this and is going through the same thing, or suspects that someone she knows is going through the same thing, can go to get help sooner.

Thankfully, Marc was not feeling as overwhelmed as I was. But then again, he got to "escape" to go to work every day. And he wasn't waking up in the middle of the night, so he wasn't sleep deprived either. And he did not have fluctuating hormones.

How long did it last? This is the part I feel really guilty about. I think it lasted, on a certain level, for two and a half years. Max was eighteen months old when Kate was born, and Kate was a full year old when I think I finally snapped out of my old being and into my new one. Do you know how some people say they had a change of heart? I think I had a change of spirit.

CG: Did something cause you to snap out of it? Or was it just a matter of time?

LL: Well, you know that feeling you have when you are not quite living an authentic life? Or when you are swimming upstream, though if you just made a few choices—sometimes difficult ones—you could swim downstream and breathe a sigh of relief? Well, somewhere deep down I knew I was not happy. My soul was not at peace. My spirit was oppressed. I know that is a strong word, and I was the one who was sort of responsible for this.

CG: You make it seem so terrible. You must not have been getting the kind of help you needed.

LL: You are right—I was not yet. And this may even be what prompted me to go back to school to become a school counselor a year later. I think I was searching for myself—for my authentic self. I was lost and trying to find myself and find my happiness.

CG: You should have read that great book called *The Happiness Project* by Gretchen Rubin.[130]

LL: Unfortunately, that book had not yet been written. I have since read it and love how the author says she was prompted to write it by her realization that "the days are long but the years are short." But in any case, I am not even sure I was out of my fog enough to be able to see that I needed a book like that—or therapy—or even the Lexapro that I later began taking to significantly cut down on all my obsessive worrying.

I know it might seem very negative and like a real low point in my life, but I don't think it was so much that. I was still functioning. I was working part time at the Internet company at that point, and I was not depressed per se, but I did get a true-blue diagnosis of anxiety, and it seems that was what was exacerbating all my worrying. I had always been a worrier and had always had anxiety, but I think that another "gift" of having children was that my hormones went haywire and made my anxiety much worse.

---

130 Gretchen Rubin, *Happiness Project* (New York: Workman, 2011).

CG: Hormones are often greatly affected by pregnancy, childbirth, nursing, and even sleep deprivation, and it sounded like you had all of these things—for two and a half years.

LL: I came to learn and really understand that so much of the spirit and soul of a mother is not in changing who you are, but rather in incorporating this new being into your life and into your definition of who you are. And then these little beings get older, and they start having thoughts that are different from yours...and ideas...and goals. This causes a whole different set of parenting issues and experiences—like the idea of thinking that our children's souls are anything like our own. Sometimes they are, but sometimes they are not. Our children are their own people with their own spirits and souls!

As a high school and middle school counselor, I am constantly honored to be part of children's inner lives, and I regularly hear about their home lives. I am also in constant contact with a very large group of parents. Most of them are very loving and wonderful, but some are not. Some try to get their children to be who they want them to be, and they sometimes don't see who they really are through their veil of who they *want* them to be. I think all parents struggle with this at some point—they think that they get this child who is a blank slate that they can shape to their liking. They find out later that this little being has her own personality and thoughts and ideas and spirit and soul, all of which are not necessarily like her mom's. This causes countless problems for the students and angst for the parents. At least once a year I send out the following quote by Khalil Gibran in my parent newsletter:

ON CHILDREN
...Your children are not your children.
They are the sons and daughters of life's longing for itself.
They come through you but not from you,
And though they are with you yet they belong not to you.
You may give them your love but not your thoughts.
For they have their own thoughts.
You may house their bodies but not their souls,
For their souls dwell in the house of tomorrow, which you cannot visit, not even in your dreams.
You may strive to be like them, but seek not to make them like you.
For life goes not backward nor tarries with yesterday...
      From *The Prophet* by Khalil Gibran

LL: Just as our parents were not able to impose *their* ideas on us and turn us into the exact people they wanted us to be, we cannot not expect our children to be who we think they should be. So why even suffer in trying? Let them figure out who they are and then support them. Meet them where they are and then go from there.

CG: Laura! I can see how it is easy to go off on a tangent about parenting when you start off with childbirth, but let's get back to vaginas!

LL: Oops. Great point. Yes, babies come out into the world, usually through our vaginas. They leave their wear and tear on our bodies, and then they are very much their own people—their own beings, their own souls. We have the honor of raising children, and we hope that their bodies are aligned with their innermost beings and souls, just like we hope that our own vaginas and feelings about our bodies are aligned with our own spirit and soul.

Suggested Resources:

Rubin, Gretchen, *Happiness Project* (New York: Workman, 2007).

Diamant, Anita, *The Red Tent* (New York: Picador, 2007).

CHAPTER 18

Sexual Orientation

LL: I am glad that we are living in a time that is *more* open to women defining themselves on their own terms and not on someone else's. It is so much easier to be in touch with your true, authentic self when you are able to define yourself, and not let others put you in a box just because it makes the most sense to them. I know that this is not true for everyone, but I am glad to see it happening more and more.

CG: Laura, as you know, it has not always been this way. For years I had a therapy practice where I saw a large number of gay, lesbian, bisexual, and other individuals, and I saw this change happening right before my eyes. When I first started my practice forty years ago, our culture was not as comfortable with homosexuality as it is today. I'm not saying we are there yet, but we are much improved. My practice was in Charlotte, and the South took a bit longer to embrace other kinds of sexual orientation than, say, many areas in California or New York. I had a lot of clients who really suffered because on the one hand, they *wanted* to be true to their inner selves and their sexual orientation, but on the other hand, they also wanted to fit in and be accepted by friends, family members, and the community, which was very heterosexual-focused and not always accepting of differences.

LL: Again, it's the whole struggle between what other people want for you and what you are—the inner voice trying to express who you really are.

CG: True. It wasn't until the 1960s that it became mainstream to even recognize sexual minorities as a group. Sexual minorities are people whose sexual identity, orientation, or practices differ from the majority of the surrounding society[131]. Initially, when it was coined in the 1960s, the term referred primarily to lesbians, gays, and bisexuals, though the majority of the focus was on the GL (gay and lesbian) part and T (transgender) was not nationally recognized until approximately 2000. These four groups are often grouped together under the category LGBT. Recently some people have added on the letter Q, which can stand for individuals who are still questioning their sexual orientation or for *queer*, which is seen as a term of endearment and not a negative word. That is why we often see the group called LGBTQ.

I like the Q for questioning because from what I saw in my practice, many women have sexual orientations that change over time. Many women (and men, too) go through stages of questioning all throughout their lives, and this is very normal.

LL: When I was doing research for this book, I read a book called *Why Women Have Sex* by Dr. Cindy M. Meston and Dr. David M. Buss. They discussed this great study where people were asked to define their sexual orientation and they found that "Eleven percent actually did not choose one of these labels [heterosexual, bisexual or homosexual] opting for "other"—including gay, lesbian, asexual, bi-curious, hetero-flexible, omnisexual, pansexual, queer, straight-plus, fluid, open, polyamorous, still questioning, and various combinations such as 'mostly heterosexual plus a touch of gay.'"[132]

---

[131] Today many people who we would consider to be sexual minorities don't even like that term because *minority* has connotations of hardship.
[132] Meston and Buss, *Why Women Have Sex: Understanding Sexual Motivations from Adventure to Revenge (and Everything in Between)*, 31.

CG: Isn't that fabulous?

LL: I say, "You go, girls" to not feeling like you have to fit into one box on the check-off list. You don't like the choices? Make up your own answer. Define yourself. I love it.

I have often wondered if women's sexual orientation is more fixed or more fluid. In the work that you did, did you draw any conclusions about whether some women are born lesbians and others have a more fluid sexuality, but find that they are more attracted to women over time?

CG: From what I have seen, I think you can't answer that question definitively. Remember, we can't put women in boxes and neat categories. There are definitely some women who are fixed, and you may say *born* lesbians. If you ever read the book *When I Knew*,[133] you will read great stories about many adults who knew they were gay when they were children. Other women are fluid. Some women are bisexual. Others are heterosexual, and then later on in life bisexual or gay. And many heterosexual women still have fantasies and sexual dreams about other women, though they were born heterosexual and define themselves as heterosexual.

There are two interesting studies highlighted on the next couple of pages that emphasize how this is not really an easy answer. The studies show that close to a fifth of women have had sexual experiences with another woman, but a much smaller percent define themselves as exclusively gay. Approximately seventeen percent of women from the Shere Hite study (compared to 19 percent in the Kinsey study) either preferred sex with women or identified as bisexual and had sexual experiences with men and women.

Alfred Kinsey and his staff at the Institute of Sex Research found that women (and men) could be described as being on a *spectrum* when it comes to sexual orientation. The spectrum ranges from zero, which represents an exclusively heterosexual response, to six, which represents an exclusively homosexual response. They found that seventy-one percent of women defined themselves as exclusively heterosexual and the remaining twenty-nine percent were anywhere from one to six on the scale. In other words, it is just too difficult to put sexual orientation into neat boxes and many, many women defy being put into neat categories. Sex researcher Fritz Klein built on this work, and he created a grid to help people figure out their sexual orientation based on their different thoughts, actions and ideals.

---

[133] Robert Trachtenberg, *When I Knew* (New York: Harper Collins, 2005).

Research on Female Sexual Orientation

The most extensive early study of female homosexuality was completed by the Institute for Sex Research, which published an in-depth report of the sexual experiences of American women in 1953. Alfred Kinsey and the staff of the Institute for Sex Research interviewed more than fifty-nine hundred women and their responses were compiled in a book titled *Sexual Behavior in the Human Female*, popularly known as part of the Kinsey Reports.[134]

Kinsey and his staff reported that twenty-eight percent of women had been aroused by another female, and nineteen percent had had sexual contact with another female. Of women who had had sexual contact with another female, one-half to two-thirds of them had orgasmed. Single women had the highest prevalence of homosexual activity, followed by women who were widowed, divorced, or separated. The lowest occurrence of sexual activity was among married women. Some of those with previous homosexual experience reported that they had gotten married to stop homosexual activity.

Most of the women who reported homosexual activity had not experienced it more than ten times. Fifty-one percent of women reporting a homosexual experience had only one partner. Women with postgraduate education had a higher prevalence of homosexual experience, followed by women with a college education. The smallest occurrence was among women with education no higher than eighth grade.

Based on Kinsey's scale where zero represents a person with an *exclusively heterosexual response* and six represents a person with an *exclusively homosexual one*, six percent of those interviewed ranked as a six—exclusively homosexual. Apart from those who ranked zero (71 percent), the largest percentage in between zero and six was one, at approximately 15 percent. However, the Kinsey Report remarked that the ranking described a period in a person's life, and that a person's orientation may change.

---

[134] Alfred C. Kinsey, et al., *Sexual Behavior in the Human Female*. (Philadelphia, PA: W.B. Saunders, 1953, 1998). See also http://www.kinseyinstitute.org/research/ak-data.html#Scope.

LL: So the Kinsey Report was mostly based on the actions the individual took. And it reported that nineteen percent of women had had sexual contact with another woman, yet only six percent were *exclusively* homosexual. Interesting. And the other thirteen percent were either bisexual, or more fluid, or experimenting, or something else. It is interesting to note here that the homosexual experience percentages are very high, despite this survey having being taken at a time in history where being gay was not as accepted by our culture.

CG: That really is fascinating. Twenty-three years after the Kinsey Report, in 1976, sexologist Shere Hite published *The Hite Report*, a report on the sexual encounters of 3,019 women who had responded to questionnaires. Hite's questions differed from Kinsey's, focusing more on how women identified or what they *preferred*, rather than on their *experiences*. Respondents to Hite's questions indicated that eight percent preferred sex with women and an additional nine percent identified as bisexual or had sexual experiences with men and women though they refused to indicate a preference. Hite's conclusions are based more on respondents' comments than on quantifiable data. She found it "striking" that many women who had had no lesbian experiences indicated that they were interested in sex with women, particularly because the question was not even asked. Hite found that the two most significant differences between respondents' experiences with men and women were the focus on clitoral stimulation, and more emotional involvement and orgasmic responses. Since Hite performed her study during the peak of feminism's popularity in the 1970s, she also acknowledged that women might have chosen to identify as lesbian for political reasons.[135]

LL: Fascinating. Now I can see how it looks like some women have a more fixed sexual orientation while others are more fluid.

And now I have a big question that I am hoping you can answer for me. If almost one in five women is not purely heterosexual—and maybe this is even higher—then why do so many women suffer coming to terms with their sexual orientation? I don't want to sound naïve, but this is a very large percentage, so why are we as a culture not super comfortable with it?

CG: Well…this is not an easy answer. In short, things just take time. Change takes time. Just as our Vagina Revolution is going to take time, this will take time. You know, in my day women were not nearly as comfortable speaking about breasts as they are now. But then along came public health campaigns encouraging women to do breast exams to detect breast cancer earlier, and

---

135 Shere Hite, *The Hite Report: A Nationwide Study of Female Sexuality* (New York, NY: Seven Stories Press, 2003), 512.

now *breast* is practically a common, household term. Women and men both wear shirts that say things like Save the Ta-Tas and other references to breasts. I predict that sexual orientation will be much more accepted in my grandchildren's lifetimes. Heck, it already is about a thousand times more acceptable than it was in my day.

LL: At the same time, we should recognize that it is still harder for many sexual minorities. People who identify as gay, lesbian, bisexual, or transgender have higher rates of stress, anxiety, and depression, as well as more suicidal ideation and a higher rate of suicide. I studied this in counseling graduate school and was shocked to see how much it affects sexual minorities and kids who are sexual minorities in particular.

CG: True. And I don't want to brush over the attitudes of many Americans about homosexuality. Until very recently it was taboo. Numerous people in the United States were brought up to think that homosexuality was "bad," a "sin," or some other negative connotation. Although things are changing, there are still examples of Americans not accepting homosexuality—just look at all the bills being brought up in each state to define marriage as a relationship between a woman and a man. We do have many states in the United States where the majority of people are more accepting of sexual minorities, but also many states where they are not.

There are many examples of countries whose populations are opposed to homosexuality—or even take a stronger stance. For example, in some Middle Eastern and African countries, if you are found to be gay, you get the death penalty. I just heard a story about this on NPR recently. In Saudi Arabia, if they find out you are gay, you are executed publically. Think about the message that sends to the teenager who is sure she is gay.

LL: But of course, there are also countries that are much more accepting and progressive than we are. My husband, Marc, who is Canadian, loves to point out that gay marriage is legal, accepted, and not a big deal in Canada. In fact, if you look at a survey Pew did in 2007, seventy percent of Canadians said that "Homosexuality should be accepted by society," compared to forty-nine percent of Americans. And in case you are wondering which other countries are more accepting, eighty-six percent of Swedes, eighty-three percent in France and the Czech Republic, eighty-two percent in Spain, eighty-one percent in Germany, seventy-one percent in Britain, and sixty-five percent in Italy. I could go on and on. We Americans are more similar to the Japanese, who are at fifty percent. Only one percent of Egyptians agreed that homosexuality should be accepted by society, and six percent of Jordanians. And most other Middle

Eastern countries (except for Israel), as well as African countries are between two and four percent.

CG: The United States is definitely moving in a more progressive direction. For example, if you look at the older generation of Americans who were born between 1925-1942, called the Silent Generation, only thirty-three percent believe in marriage equity (gay and lesbian individuals being allowed to marry)—compared to fifty-nine percent of the younger Millennial Generation. Even the Silent Generation has changed its views on this over time as well—their percentage is up from twenty percent believing in marriage equity in 1996.[136]

The first state to *decriminalize* homosexuality was Illinois in 1961. The first state to pass a law to protect the rights of gays and lesbians was Wisconsin, and that was not until 1982. And get this—sodomy was not federally decriminalized until 2003.[137] In our lifetimes. You are young so you probably do not remember this one…it was not until 1973—

LL: Hey, I was five in 1973…

CG: …that the American Psychiatric Association removed homosexuality from its list of diseases.

LL: We have come a long way, baby. But we have a much longer way to go to ensure that women (and men) can feel safe to express their true sexual orientation and inner identity.

And one last thing—if you define yourself one way, but you think in some way you are changing, do not worry. I love how Dr. Lissa Rankin phrases this when she talks about this topic in her book *What's Up Down There*.

> "Most important, how do you identify yourself? It's not whether other women turn you on, who you fantasize about, or even how you behave. It's how you feel inside. As you grow older, your sexuality may evolve. Don't be afraid of how you feel.
>
> "If you know deep down that you're bisexual or a lesbian, you may be scared to acknowledge these feelings because you fear isolation, loss of friends and family, and other societal conflicts, which may be very real. If you feel confused or ashamed, or you're in the process of coming out,

---

[136] "Views on Social Issues by Generation," Pew Research Center, November 11, 2011, accessed September 2012, http://www.pewresearch.org/daily-number/views-on-social-issues-by-generation/.

[137] *Lawrence v. Texas* 539 U.S. 558 (2003).

consider talking to a counselor who can help you work through your feelings."[138]

CG: As a practitioner, I have seen women of every different orientation, and I have been honored to be with them when they explore their sexual orientations — which sometimes changes over time. These are very soulful explorations, and they are often filled with emotion. There is a very powerful connection between a woman's feelings about her vagina and her body, her sexual orientation, and how she defines herself in general.

LL: I hope that the more women feel comfortable with their vaginas and bodies, the more in line they can be with their souls and their authentic selves.

Join the Revolution! **Be True to Your Sexual Orientation.**

We are socialized by our families and communities, and many of us have felt the need to repress natural feelings in order to fit in or be accepted by loved ones. Yet when you repress real, natural feelings, those feelings don't sit back and take it for very long because they have a strong need to get out and get recognized. And why wouldn't they if they are real and authentic? If you have not already paid attention to those feelings and ideas, then do so now. Brought up learning to like men, but really attracted to women? Explore this idea. Have fantasies and dreams about being a lesbian? They may not actually mean you are a lesbian. Or maybe they do. Sexuality is very fluid — more so for women than for men, and even more so over time. No matter what the thoughts and feelings, explore them now or when the time is right.

We all have a right to define ourselves in whatever way we want to.

Suggested Resources:

Berzon, Betty, *Permanent Partners: Building Gay and Lesbian Relationships that Last* (New York: Plume, 1990).

Clark, Don H, *Loving Someone Gay* (Maple Shade, NJ: Lethe, 2009).

---

[138] Rankin, *What's Up Down There? Questions You'd Only Ask Your Gynecologist If She Was Your Best Friend*, 116.

Diamond, Lisa M, *Sexual Fluidity: Understanding Women's Love and Desire* (Cambridge, MA: Harvard University Press, 2009).

Loulan, Joann, *Lesbian Sex* (San Francisco, CA: Spinsters Ink Books, 1984).

Loulan, Joann, *Lesbian Passion: Loving Ourselves* (San Francisco, CA: Aunt Lute Books, 1987).

McNaught, Brian R, *On Being Gay: Thoughts on Family, Faith and Love* (New York: St. Martin's Press, 1986).

Weinberg, Martin S., Colin J. Williams and Douglas W. Pryor, *Dual Attraction: Understanding Bisexuality* (New York: Oxford University Press, 1995).

Kinsey, Alfred C. et al, *Sexual Behavior in the Human Female* (Philadelphia, PA: W.B. Saunders, 1953, 1998) [Discusses the Kinsey Scale and presents comparisons of male and female data, see 468–475.]

Klein, Fritz et al., "Sexual Orientation: A Multi-Variable Dynamic Process," *Journal of Homosexuality*, 11, 1–2 (1985): 35–49. [Discusses the problem of lack of clear, widely accepted definitions of heterosexual, bisexual, and homosexual].

Sell, Randall L, "The Sell Assessment of Sexual Orientation: Background and Scoring," *Journal of Gay, Lesbian, and Bisexual Identity*, 1, 4 (1996): 295–310. [Includes review of sexual orientation measures, which are characterized as dichotomous, bipolar, multidimensional, and/or orthogonal.]

CHAPTER 19

Gender Identity

CG: Transgender individuals are often lumped in with gay, lesbian, bisexual, and questioning individuals, and it is true that all of these individuals share some challenges in common, but there are also so many differences.

Perhaps because there are more people who are gay, lesbian, and bisexual, society understands this more. It is harder in some ways to understand the challenges that gender identity has for many people. I will try to explain this.

Our culture has one *main* way about thinking about gender. Each child is assigned a sex at birth—either male or female. *If you have a vagina, you are a girl, and if you have a penis, you are a boy*. And our culture spends a lot of time and energy teaching children to accept and celebrate these two very distinct categories. But many individuals feel like this categorization goes against what they feel inside. Many individuals feel that their assigned sex does not match their gender or gender identity.

> Gender identity is a person's private sense of, and subjective experience of, their own gender. If you were assigned the sex female when you were born and you always felt like the roles assigned to females fit your personality, then you probably would have no reason to question anything—just as the last thing a fish notices is water.
>
> Just because a person is born with a vagina, that does not mean the person wants to fit into the narrowly defined classification that we have come to think of in our culture as female. And if a person is born with a penis but at the most soulful level wants a vagina and wants to be a woman, then why shouldn't she?

One of the first concepts a young child learns is that people are divided into two different sexes—male and female—and the child learns that she is a girl or he is a boy. Our culture has a *binary* view of gender—you are *either* a boy *or* a girl.

Most societies in recent recorded history have been set up to encourage us—either through conformity (or rather punishment if we don't conform)—to acknowledge and adopt the ideals of masculinity and femininity in all aspects of gender and sex. This includes gender identity, gender expression, and biological sex.

LL: I remember asking my older son, when he was just learning to talk, how he could tell if someone was a boy or a girl—and he said the typical "Girls have long hair and boys don't."

CG: That is so classic. I think one of my kids said that, too. And there is something to be said about that—many women hold their femininity in their long hair.

LL: And then the next level in our house was just like in the movie *Kindergarten Cop*: "Boys have penises, and girls have vaginas." I remember vividly one day when my niece Eden was about three, and she looked around in the car and said, "Hey! We all have vaginas!" There were five of us in the car, and yep, we were all female.

CG: Gender identity is so accentuated when kids are young. Just as we assimilate our children into our culture by emphasizing our values and enforcing our rules, we also reinforce gender stereotypes in so many conscious and unconscious ways. For example, when teachers divide the class into boys and girls; when we allow our boys to be more aggressive and tell our girls not to be; when we ooh and ah over our daughter's dresses and hairstyles, but applaud our sons for running fast. People just do this as second nature. Most of the time we don't think twice about any of this.

I know when I was younger and raising my kids that I didn't give this a lot of thought.

LL: But if you had a different gender identity, or if you had recently had a patient who did, then you would probably be hyperaware of all of this. I put a lot of stock in gender identity issues because of what I studied in counseling graduate school but even more because of what I saw as a school counselor. Some of my students experienced distress with their assigned gender, and it caused some havoc in their lives. I had one student who did not seem to experience much distress, and he was very proud of who he was. It made me feel so good to see him comfortable in his own skin. He was born with all of the male characteristics but in ninth grade, the only year he was at my school, he only ever dressed as a female, and he insisted on using the girls bathroom. The school administration did not let him, but he felt so strongly that I know he snuck in there anyway.

In my experiences as a school counselor, in counseling graduate school, and through research, I have found that the whole binary view of gender—that a person is *either* female *or* male—is actually too simple. My friends don't really get this when I try to explain it, but it makes complete sense to me.

I found that there are some cultures today in Asia, and there have been others throughout history that are less binary-sex-focused. For example, in India, there is a "third gender" or "third sex." This describes individuals who are categorized by their will or by social consensus as *neither man nor woman*. Some sociologists and anthropologists even describe four, five, or more genders.

CG: Do you really think there could be five separate genders?

LL: I think there could be more than that. I would define a person's gender as *whatever his or her self-definition is*, and I think that is a matter of how she or he feels in her or his soul. *Gender identity* is very much dependent on the person, and whether or not the person defines him- or herself as a male or female, or neither, or both, or any other way. If there is a contrast between how I define my identity and how others assign my identity, then this will likely make me feel bad and I would experience conflict in my soul.

CG: So what I hear you saying is that gender identity comes from the soul.

LL: Yes. And when someone's soul is aligned with her body and feelings about her body, she can feel comfortable in her own skin. But if the two are misaligned, this causes many people to feel shame when they are labeled something different than what they feel.

This is much more common than you might think. In fact, a survey of research literature from 1955 to 2000 suggests that as many as two in every hundred individuals may have some intersex characteristic.[139] Intersex is defined as human beings whose biological sex cannot be classified as clearly male or female.

CG: Do you mean like transgender men and women?

LL: Transgender is a general term applied to a variety of individuals, behaviors, and groups that tend to vary from culturally conventional gender roles. So transgender is the state of one's gender identity (self-identification as a woman, man, neither, or both) not matching one's assigned sex (identification by others as male, female or intersex—based on physical or genetic sex).

CG: The definition sounds a bit confusing.

LL: There was another school counselor in my school district who could serve as a great example of what I mean. Renya was born Robert, but she always felt like a woman. Although she dressed and presented as a man at work, she dressed and presented as a female in her personal life. I met her when she was on a panel of transgender people who came to talk to my graduate school class called Counseling Sexual Minorities. She said if she could do it over she would have gone through gender reassignment surgery when she was younger. She was close to sixty years old and said that in her younger days she had been too afraid of being ostracized. So instead she chose to hide who she really was during the day.

---

139 Melanie Blackless, Anthony Charuvastra, Amanda Derryck, Anne Fausto-Sterling, Karl Lauzanne, and Ellen Lee, "How Sexually Dimorphic Are We? Review and Synthesis." *American Journal of Human Biology* 12 (2): 151–166, accessed July 9, 2012, http://www.ncbi.nlm.nih.gov/pubmed/11534012.

CG: That must not have felt very good—to have to hide who you really are. There is no chance of being authentic in every aspect.

LL: It is so difficult to be truly authentic for anyone let alone someone who feels like she has to hide her true gender. And to get back to the topic of our book—can you imagine being born with a vagina and not wanting one because in your soul you feel like you are a man, and you should have a penis? Or can you imagine being born with a penis but always feeling like you should have a vagina? I think for some people this would be very difficult to imagine, but I know there are many individuals for whom this is a very real issue.

CG: Since this can be a bit confusing can you please try defining the terms better?

> <u>Intersex</u>
>
> Some individuals are born with chromosomes that do not correspond with their body's appearance. If a baby is born and on the outside the baby appears like a girl—the baby has a vagina and no penis, for example—then the baby is declared a girl. But there is a chance that the baby's chromosomes say something different. If someone had analyzed the baby's chromosomes at birth, they might have seen that the baby had XY (male) chromosomes and *not* XX (female), even though the baby's outward appearance looked like a girl.
>
> An intersex individual may also have biological characteristics of *both* male and female sexes. In other words, the individual may have both a penis and a vagina. In the past, a doctor either consulted with the parents or acted on her own to decide which gender the child was going to be, and then did surgery to "correct" the child. This resulted in many tragic stories where the doctor did not guess correctly, and the child ended up in the wrong gender body. Now doctors can check chromosomes or wait to do surgery until the child gives some kind of indication of his or her gender.
>
> Historically, individuals who were born with ambiguous genitalia were called *hermaphrodites*, but this term is now considered to be misleading and stigmatizing, and therefore the term *intersex* is preferred. Again, intersex is a broad term applied to human beings whose biological sex cannot be classified as clearly male or female.

> ### *Androgyny*
>
> Some people (whether physically intersex or not) do not identify themselves as either exclusively female or exclusively male. Androgyny is sometimes used to refer to those without gender-specific physical sexual characteristics, sexual orientation, gender identity or some combination of these. Androgynous individuals are people who can be physically and psychologically anywhere between the two sexes. This is not considered to be an intersex condition.
>
> ### *Transgender*
>
> The simplest way to define transgender is to say that it is someone who is born one gender but feels like another gender on the soul level. He or she may or may not have DNA to support this. The term transgender has evolved over the years it was originally used in 1965, and it has at one point or another either included transsexuals, bi-gender, cross-dressers, and others. Some transgender people seek out medical help so they can look and feel more like the gender they associate with. In other words if a man at his soul level feels like a woman, he can get hormone therapy to become more like a woman. He can also get sexual reassignment surgery. Some transgender people choose to dress like a different gender but not to get hormone therapy or sexual reassignment surgery. This is sometimes because they can't afford it or because of other medical issues or age that might make the hormones or surgery risky.

CG: I bet most people have no idea that every day they probably come into contact with people who are gender variant. And I had no idea that intersex individuals made up such a large percentage of the population—two out of every hundred people!

LL: Yes. Sometimes these individuals get diagnosed with *gender identity disorder*, but as a counselor, I cannot agree with this terminology because I do not see it as a disorder. I did just hear that the American Psychological Association is considering changing the name from disorder to *dysphoria* or *incongruence* when they come out with their next version of the Diagnostic and Statistical

Manual of Mental Disorders (DSM-V)[140]. I think that is more appropriate. I prefer to see it as a "scrambling" of categories. As humans, we tend to like neat categories so we can feel a better sense of control over our world. For example, if I know that the stranger that I'm about to meet is a woman, my subconscious can quickly calculate a lot of things about her. It doesn't mean that those things are right. That is just how our brains like to operate.

If a person defines herself as a woman although she does not have a vagina, it is only fair that we take her for her word and call her what she wants to be called—a woman. If a person has a vagina and calls himself a man, then we should follow suit.

Gender is a concept, and it is something that we *learn*. Babies aren't really *born* with a gender. They may be assigned a *sex* at birth, but they *learn* gender. Our culture reinforces gender stereotypes, and we go along with this because we are taught to. For example, when my younger son was two he picked up a tinker toy and pretended it was a gun. He had not learned this at school, and he had never seen his parents or older brother or sister do it. But we all reacted with "Oh, Charlie is such a *boy*." People like to perpetuate stereotypes so we all nod our heads and agree.

When we get older, we assume that what we learned as part of our culture is *the truth*, when in fact a lot of it just started as someone's opinion until our parents or communities believed it, went along with it, and taught it to us. Again, "the last thing a fish would ever notice would be water," and it is very difficult to change the things that we learned to be true when we were growing up.

CG: It is certainly difficult to wrap your head around if you are not used to the idea. But as a medical professional, a general rule I have is to always believe what the patient tells me. If she is feeling certain symptoms, then she has the symptoms. So if she tells me she is one gender and looks like another, then of course I will treat her as the gender she wants to be treated…but also talk to her about the medical conditions of the other gender if she has those parts. For example, if a transgender man comes to me and still has a vagina and ovaries and a uterus, I will still do a pap smear or any medical tests based on both the parts he does have and the gender identity he is.

---

140 I still do not think that just because someone defines herself differently from how others define her she should be diagnosed with a mental disorder, but I understand that if someone is transgender and is having distress because of this then she or he needs some kind of diagnosis for health insurance to pay for psychological counseling or any kind of hormone therapy or gender reassignment surgery. So for practical reasons there may be a case for keeping some kind of diagnosis in the DSM-V.

LL: Many intersex or transgender women are born without vaginas but want to have a vagina. Similarly, many transgender women do not want the penis they were born with and do want a vagina. There are more options now than ever before for going through hormone therapy or surgeries to become more in line with the gender of your identity. This is all about allowing people to feel more aligned with their souls.

One thing I find particularly fascinating about this is when a woman wants to create a vagina where there was not one previously. Do you know that through hormones and surgeries, doctors can remove a penis and surgically create a vagina?

I think it is amazing, partly because of the medical lengths that individuals go through to have their body be more aligned with how they feel inside. I think it is brave and courageous to do this. But it is also amazing because it is a modern medical miracle—the creation of a vagina.

With a lot of care, including regular stretching out of the vaginal walls, a woman with a new vagina can enjoy sex, intimacy, and even orgasms.

LL: The bottom line of gender identity is that there are so, so many ways to define your gender and that gender is not necessarily binary. If your assigned or assumed gender does not feel right to you, then it is important to explore this so your gender can be more in line with your soul.

Remaining Issue of Social Justice

In the previous chapter we mentioned that the American Psychological Association (APA) still considered being gay and lesbian a mental illness until 1973. Forty years after this, in the year 2013, transgender and other gender identity issues are still given a diagnosis that is in the DSM-IV, which means that they are all still considered to be a mental illness.

Additionally, the repeal of the United State's military's Don't Ask, Don't Tell policy recently included people who were gay and lesbian but not transgendered. There are still transgender individuals being honorably discharged from the military simply because they are transgender.

Being transgender does not constitute a psychiatric disorder. A majority of transgender individuals or individuals who have other gender identity issues are healthy and well-adjusted people and do not have any mental illness. Perhaps it is only a matter of how society defines this. Perhaps if society took a broader approach to defining individuals than a simple binary view that everyone is either male or female, this would not even be an issue. Perhaps this will change in the next decade or two—our culture will recognize a broad spectrum of transgender and other gender identities, and this will not be considered a mental illness but rather just a respectable difference.

Suggested Resources:

Bachman, Barbara. *Our Bodies, Ourselves for the New Century: A Book by and for Women*. Boston Women's Health Collective, 4th ed. New York: Touchstone, 2005.

There is a great section on gender identity in this book.

Bem, Sandra Lipsitz, *The Lenses of Gender: Transforming the Debate on Sexual Inequality* (New Haven, CT: Yale University Press, 1993).

National Center for Transgender Equality website http://transequality.org/federal_gov.html.

Public Radio Exchange (PRX.org)

PRX.org is an online marketplace for public radio programming. They have many excellent radio programs on intersex and transgender issues. http://www.prx.org/search/pieces?q=transgender&x=0&y=0

Trans, the Movie. A fabulous, informative movie.

World Professional Association for Transgender Health.

This association publishes the *International Journal of Transgenderism*, and anyone can download articles free of charge by going to this link: http://www.wpath.org/journal/index.html.

CHAPTER 20

What Is Going On With Our Sisters Worldwide

"I believe that the rights of women and girls are the unfinished business of the twenty-first century…As long as girls and women are valued less, fed less, fed last, overworked, underpaid, not schooled, subjected to violence in and outside their homes—the potential of the human family to create a peaceful, prosperous world will not be realized."

Hillary Clinton, *Newsweek*, March 14, 2011

"Although the world is full of suffering, it is full also of the overcoming of it."
Helen Keller

Where I Am Coming From:

LL: OK, so I am a feminist. I believe that all women everywhere should have the same political, economic, and social rights as men. I think women should have equal opportunities in education and employment. I am wholeheartedly a supporter of the rights and equality of women — and of every person, for that matter.

But I also don't want to sound naïve in my discussion below of what is going on with our sisters worldwide — both in the United States and other countries. I am a mom, a public high school and middle school counselor, and a former policy wonk. I am not a professor, a philosopher, an activist, or up on every article from the *Atlantic* or other intellectual magazines or newspapers. I am envious of the individuals who are. But I am doing the best I can to raise three children and work outside the home, and I recognize that I cannot do everything.

But I do think that the fate of all women everywhere is very much intertwined, so I am going to point out a few things going on worldwide that I find very worrisome. They relate to bad things that are happening to vaginas. And I'm going to take the discussion to the website www.vaginarevolution.com (blog) or direct the conversation to other websites. I don't think any one person can have all the answers to these issues, but I do have confidence that when women put their heads together, they come up with effective solutions to problems. It is my hope that some readers can help with this.

Women Are Lucky to Be Women

Women are such special beings — we are so lucky to have complex systems that help us give birth to the beings we love and who help carry on the human race. We have such a wide range of feelings and such depth of emotions. We carry so much love in our hearts and guilt in our heads. We really are so complex. We want what is best for our children, our loved ones, ourselves. Most of us want world peace. We want safety and security, health and happiness for children everywhere.

And just as Eve Ensler said, "Girls literally hold the future in their bodies. People don't seem to realize that the stronger our girls are, the stronger humanity becomes."

> We women are so fortunate to have other women in our lives. Who comforts us when we lose a loved one? Who would organize a meal train when we have a baby or a chemo-buddy group so we don't have to sit alone for hours' worth of chemotherapy? Who else could pick us up when feeling down after a bad breakup? We track each other's bodies and know when we lose or gain weight, and when we are glowing or declining. We fight and then we make up and go on to be that much stronger. These women are our friends, our sisters, our daughters, our mothers, aunts, grandmothers, and colleagues. Other women give our lives infinite meaning.

Worldwide, including in our own country, many women's spirits and souls are being crushed because of their life circumstances. An estimated one million girls worldwide enter the sex trade every year, and four million women and girls are trafficked every year. A study in Nigeria found that sixteen percent of patients hospitalized for sexually transmitted infections were under the age of five. So-called "honor killings" take the lives of thousands of young women every year, especially in North Africa, western Asia, and parts of South Asia. Twenty-two million American women have been raped[141]. These statistics are only the tip of the iceberg when discussing violence against women worldwide.

I ask for you to momentarily put yourselves in the shoes of these women who are suffering. As women, we are so good at feeling empathy, feeling it deeply in our souls. And as women, we are also good at something else—seeking out the truth, knowing right from wrong, and recognizing when something needs to change. And what else are we fabulous at? Organizing to make those changes happen.

This is why I included this section of the book. It is my hope and prayer that we can see this suffering worldwide and then commit to putting an end to it.

Mutilated Vaginas
CG: No!

LL: Yes!

---

[141] These statistics are from excellent, reliable sources gathered by the feminist.com website, accessed January 2013, http://www.feminist.com/antiviolence/facts.html#global.

CG: You *cannot* bring the topic of female genital mutilation into this book. You can't bring such a negative, gruesome topic into such a positive, uplifting book.

LL: I can't help it. It's something everyone needs to know about. And I know women would *want* to know about it. Just as I love to say, "You're only as happy as your least happy child," so it is true that *women are only as happy as our least happy vagina*. In other words, if women are suffering in some places in the world, then we are all suffering on a very fundamental level.

CG: But women do know about female genital mutilation. It is on our collective radar screen. I mean, there are magazine articles about it…newspaper articles…it's in *Time* and *Newsweek*, and even in *Vogue* and other women's magazines. I even heard a story about it last week on NPR.

LL: I thought most women knew about it, too. But then I went to my girls' weekend last January and started talking about FGM to three of my closest friends Beth, Debbie, and Becky, all of whom are very educated and knowledgeable. One is a doctor in Atlanta, one is a lawyer-turned-writer in Atlanta, and one has a doctorate in psychology and is a practicing psychologist in D.C. And all three of them had no idea what I was talking about.

CG: Really?

LL: Absolutely. And they are well read, active in book clubs, local politics, and religious institutions. They all have kids and regular conversations with other mothers and husbands and neighbors. Yet they had not heard about it.

CG: Wow. Well, I do think it is important to mention, if you think other educated and caring women don't know about it. But you wouldn't consider pictures for this section, right?

LL: Wrong. Of course we need pictures for this section. It is one thing to talk about female genital mutilation (FGM), and it is another thing to show FGM — to show the results of the mutilation.

Female genital mutilation[142] is the removal of part or all of the external female genitalia. In its most severe form a woman or girl has all of her genitalia removed and then stitched together, leaving a small opening for intercourse and menstruation. It is practiced in twenty-eight countries, as well as other communities around the world (including in some immigrant communities in the United States and Canada), though it is heavily concentrated in Africa and

---

[142] Definition from Amnesty International, accessed November 2012, http://www.amnestyusa.org/our-work/issues/women-s-rights/violence-against-women/violence-against-women-information.

the Middle East. Over two million girls every year are subjected to FGM, and an estimated one hundred and thirty-five million girls and women have undergone FGM worldwide.

FGM is often done in unsanitary conditions, often with barbers doing the cutting. And there is a long list of medical complications that come along with FGM, ranging from infection to sterility to death. FGM also causes complications in childbirth and increased risk of newborn deaths.

FGM is mostly carried out on young girls between infancy and fifteen years old. Girls are often not told what the procedure is going to be like, and it is usually done against their will.

The world has recognized that this should end—in 2008, the World Health Organization (WHO) came out with a statement that FGM should be eliminated. Many countries have made the practice illegal on paper but they do not enforce the law and as a result FGM continues to thrive.

Here is a picture of the vagina of someone who has gone through FGM. You cannot see that her clitoris has been removed because after removing the clitoris and inner labia, her outer labia were sewn together so that there is only room for her urine and menstrual blood to come out.

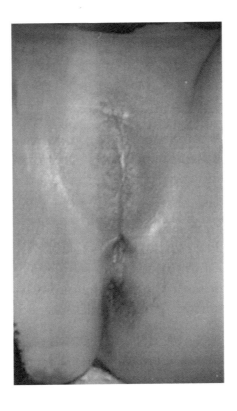

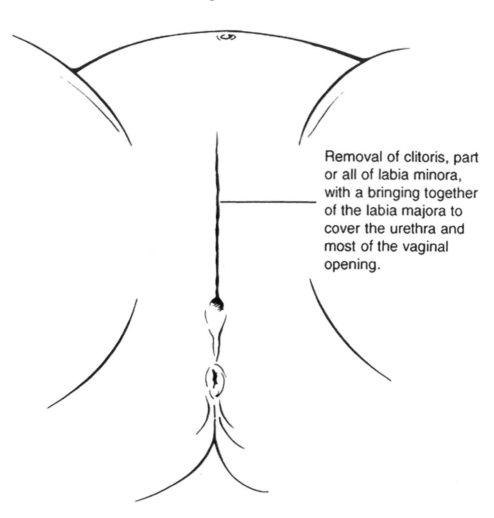

Removal of clitoris, part or all of labia minora, with a bringing together of the labia majora to cover the urethra and most of the vaginal opening.

There are different levels of FGM. In some countries and some cultures part or all of the clitoris is removed, but the labia are not sewn together. The picture above[143] is what is called Type III FGM, and the diagram above is from an article in the American Academy of Pediatrics[144]

One thing that makes me angry about FGM is that people in many societies and cultures cut off part or all of a girl's vulva and clitoris so that she will be "pure" and not want to have sex because she can't feel pleasure. Not only is the practice dangerous, but it assumes that vaginas and sex are dirty and impure. When women who have undergone FGM get married, they experience a great deal of pain as their husband has to break through the scar tissue that has

---

143 Thank you to the website www.Middle-East-Info.org for giving us permission to reprint this photo and diagram. http://www.middle-east-info.org/league/somalia/fgmpictures.htm.

144 *Pediatrics*, vol. 102, 1 (1998) : 153-156.

formed after the FGM. Sometimes women have to have an additional surgery just to open up their labia. Sadly women cannot experience as much sexual pleasure because they do not have a clitoris, and there is a great deal of scar tissue left over from the FGM. This usually causes lifelong problems.

CG: I know that FGM is horrible and painful. In some cultures, though, it is entirely accepted. It is not called *female genital mutilation* but rather *female circumcision*. In some cultures in Africa and in some Middle Eastern countries, if a woman doesn't go through these…procedures…she is shunned by the community. She can't find a husband and has no way of making money. It can be like a death sentence. I know it sounds cruel and gruesome and wrong…but on the other hand, who are we to go to another culture and tell them what to do? Who are we to tell a council of women in Liberia or Kenya or Egypt that an age-old custom that they lived through, and their aunts and mothers and grandmothers took part in, should just end?

LL: And who were we to tell Hitler to stop murdering Jews and so many others? It wasn't our country. Who were we to tell South Africa to end apartheid? Or Britain to end its occupation of India? Why should we tell a leader of another country what they should do?

But maybe my language is harsh and therefore ineffective. I have to change my vocabulary here because you are right on one level. We should not necessarily *tell* another culture what to do — no one wants to be told — but there are already feminist activists in these cultures working toward positive change. They are in the minority, but we can support them and their efforts to help *the citizens* make the changes in their cultures and countries.

CG: I like that much better.

LL: Throughout time, humans have engaged in practices that were inhumane and immoral. Over time, they have ended, one by one. It was extremely common to sacrifice human babies thousands of years ago. Or to stone to death a teenager who was not obeying an elder. Or even in more recent history — in our own Charlotte, North Carolina, a eugenics board forty years ago routinely sterilized adults whom they did not deem "fit to bear and raise children."

CG: I've heard about that in the news lately. I think the North Carolina legislature has voted to compensate those victims by giving them fifty thousand dollars each.

LL: The ones who are alive. Many have died. But it was completely immoral for social workers and state legislators to decide who was going to be sterilized.

Many of those individuals did not have power or rights, and something bad was done to them as a result. That is immoral.

CG: But who defines morality? I mean we did that to people in our own country—rather, our own state and city—and then the policy was determined to be inhumane, and it ended. What if Saudi Arabia had told us from afar in 1950 that what we were doing was extremely wrong? Would we have listened? Would that have been fair?

LL: *I wish they had told us.* And I wish they had found the activists in our state who were fighting against this—assuming there were activists fighting this issue at the time. Or at least I wish they had attempted to end those practices by pressuring us through the court of public opinion. People have a *moral authority* and *moral imperative* to try to change something that they think is wrong.

But let me back up for a minute. Every situation needs to be taken on a case-by-case basis. I do think that people in every country have the moral authority to look at what is going on within their country and outside their country and identify when something is wrong. The United Nations does this all of the time. And **every** country has done things that have been wrong—all peoples in all cultures—since the beginning of time. But as we evolve and learn to tell good from bad, right from wrong, we need to make rules, laws, guidelines, and suggestions, and we need to do whatever is in our power to help others. And yes, you are right, it is best to support the individuals who are making progress in their own communities, cultures, and countries.

Here is an example:

Every woman and man has the *moral authority* to stand up for what is right.

There are no borders when we are standing up for others. When the United States put Japanese individuals in internment camps in the 1940s, it was wrong and immoral. A majority of the Japanese people were American citizens. Many people in the United States realized that this was wrong, and it even became a case before the Supreme Court in 1944, and our very own Supreme Court held up the order. In 1988 Congress passed and President Reagan signed into legislation an apology to our own Japanese-American citizens, but this was too little, too

> late, just as it was too late to reverse forced sterilizations performed on North Carolinian citizens in the 1960s and 1970s.
>
> And then look at what the Japanese did around that same time. The Japanese military captured and kidnapped hundreds of thousands of women from China, Korea, Japan, and the Philippines and forced them to be sexual slaves. Some of the women and girls were daughters of their enemies, and some were literally lied to and kidnapped. The military set up "comfort stations" where military men could go to *rape* these "comfort women." These women were certainly not the ones getting any comfort. Instead most of them died, became infertile, or got sexually transmitted infections. Those who did survive likely never got over the trauma of being sexual slaves. The Japanese government has given a half-hearted apology for what happened and has also paid reparations to women from South Korea. However, the surviving women for the most part are not satisfied that the Japanese government has taken responsibility for what happened.

CG: There are stories of horrible and immoral things done to people and women in every country in the past and even today.

LL: It is true. I've put a list of examples of what is still going on today in the appendices, and I also put a link on the vaginarevolution.com website.[145] The information was taken from the Amnesty International fact sheet titled "Making Violence Against Women Count." The sad thing is that we can't even call this history because it is still happening at this very moment.

But back to mutilated vaginas. I know this is not an entirely black and white issue. I mean, to me it feels black and white because I was brought up in a different culture and not in the culture where it was the norm.

But putting culture aside (though I know this is impossible to do), **the bottom line of FGM is that female health and sexuality is diminished because of the**

---

[145] Amnesty International Fact Sheet, "Violence Against Women," *Amnesty International*, n.d., accessed January 11, 2013, http://www.amnestyusa.org/our-work/issues/women-s-rights/violence-against-women/violence-against-women-information.

perceived needs of men. It is patriarchy personified — patriarchy being defined as a society in which male members predominate in positions of power.

This is recognized widely:

> "It is indisputable that the woman is not just being maimed anatomically, but also that her sexual function is being impaired. Worse still, nearly all analyses of the purpose of this custom show that the main motive is the subjection of female sexuality to the perceived needs of men."[146]

Furthermore, "FGM is recognized internationally as a violation of the human rights of girls and women. It reflects deep-rooted inequality between the sexes, and constitutes an extreme form of discrimination against women. It is nearly always carried out on minors and is a violation of the rights of children. The practice also violates a person's rights to health, security, and physical integrity, the right to be free from torture and cruel, inhuman or degrading treatment, and the right to life when the procedure results in death."[147]

Despite opposition from WHO, UNICEF, and thousands of other nonprofits and agencies, FGM is still practiced in twenty-eight countries worldwide.[148] In some countries — like Egypt, for example — ninety-one percent of married women aged fifteen to forty-nine have undergone female genital mutilation.[149]

CG: If there are such strong advocates on both sides of the issue, that really indicates that there is much more here than meets the eye.

LL: This is where the questions come in that I referred to earlier. Sometimes the answers to complicated issues are best discovered when many minds meet, especially including the minds of women who are in the culture we are debating about.

I am posing some questions here, and then I suggest taking the conversation onto www.vaginarevolution.com, as well as the other websites that are addressing these issues full time.

---

[146] Drenth, *The Origin of the World: Science and Fiction of the Vagina*, 185.
[147] World Health Organization, http://www.equalitynow.org/fgm.
[148] A, UN, 2002.
[149] WHO survey, 2008, http://www.who.int/reproductivehealth/topics/fgm/prevalence/en/index.html

Questions:

Why don't we find our own culture's practices as viscerally horrifying as foreign practices?

Do you think that the lesson of FGM can help us reflect on the ways violence is normalized in our own culture?

Have you ever considered extreme dieting or wearing stilettos or facelifts as a kind of violence that women inflict upon themselves?

What do women do in our culture to be seen as being fully or properly *feminine*? For example, shaving one's legs or underarms, wearing a bra, styling one's hair, dieting, or getting a breast job?

Does our culture have harmful, painful customs for transforming bodies into "normally gendered bodies"?

Do you think that women need to appear or act more feminine to get what they want like a partner or a job?

Rape and Sexual Violence

LL: FGM is only one form of violence that is regularly practiced against girls and women. There are many other forms of violence, too. For example, rape is the most violent form of sexual violence. Rape is also associated with unwanted pregnancies and sexually transmitted infections. However, rape is greatly underreported because of the stigma attached to it, and even more rarely punished. It is probably the most underreported crime in the United States.

It is estimated that **globally one out of three women will be beaten, coerced into sex, have some kind of trauma to their vaginas, or otherwise be abused in their lifetimes, with rates reaching seventy percent in some countries.**[150] The United States and other Western countries are not immune to this.

In the United States, nearly one in five women surveyed said they had been raped or had experienced an attempted rape at some point, and one in four reported having been beaten by an intimate partner.[151] To make this seem

---

[150] World Health Organization, Multi-Country Study on Women's Health and Domestic Violence against Women, 2005.
[151] Roni Caryn Rabin, "Nearly 1 in 5 Women in US Survey Say They Have Been Sexually Assaulted, *New York Times*, 2011.

more urgent, listen to this — in the United States, a woman is raped every ninety seconds.[152]

LL: Violence within the family (also known as domestic violence) is also a problem in the United States and worldwide. Many women suffer from physical aggression such as slapping, hitting, kicking, and beating (physical abuse), as well as psychological abuse such as intimidation, constant belittling, and humiliation. It's also abuse when a partner tries to control a woman by isolating her from her family and friends, monitoring and restricting her movements, and denying her access to information or assistance.

The United States, like all countries, sees its fair share of violence in the family. Usually, the abuser is a member of the woman's own family or someone known to her.[153] Additionally, up to seventy percent of female murder victims worldwide are killed by their male partners[154]

These statistics really make me want to cry. Several well-known and trustworthy organizations worldwide have found similar survey results. The National Organization of Women in the United States found that in the United States alone, more than six hundred women every day are raped or sexually assaulted, three women every day are murdered by an intimate partner, and 4.8 million women suffer from domestic violence each year.[155]

Our sisters in other countries are suffering from similar offenses:

- In Egypt, 35 percent of women reported being beaten by their husband at some point in their marriage (UNICEF 2000).
- In Canada, the costs of violence against the family amount to $1.6 billion per year, including medical care and lost productivity (UNICEF 2000).
- In New Zealand, 20 percent of women reported being hit or physically abused by a male partner (UNICEF 2000).

CG: OK, not to stereotype my gender here because I know I'll get dinged for it from all corners, but as a woman, I just cannot wrap my mind around all of this violence. It just does not make sense to me, and it is hard to understand.

---

[152] U.S. Department of Justice, *National Crime Victimization Survey* (Washington, DC: GPO, 2000).

[153] L. Heise, M. Ellsberg and M. Gottemoeller, "Ending Violence Against Women," *Population Reports*, Series L, no. 11 (Baltimore, MD : John Hopkins, December 1999).

[154] World Health Organization, Multi-Country Study on Women's Health and Domestic Violence against Women, 2002.

[155] "Violence Against Women in the US: Statistics," *National Organization for Women*, n.d., accessed January 11, 2013, http://www.now.org/issues/violence/stats.html.

LL: You are lucky; you probably grew up in a peaceful home with a peaceful family, and you grew up in a relatively peaceful time in a relatively peaceful country. But many women are not so lucky. Many women live in places or families where conditions are not as safe, and rape and violence are prevalent. And many women live in countries where the laws are stacked against them.

Also, *rape culture* plays a very large role in rape and sexual violence, and our country is not immune from this. Most countries are ruled by men, and we live in patriarchal societies where men have written most of the rules and have most of the power. Now, I am not saying that times and conditions have not changed a great deal in some countries, nor am I saying that all men are bad and purposely create unfair conditions for women. But the patterns of power create very complex conditions for women and, if we look at the statistics, we can see that the conditions of power result in something being very wrong.

Have you heard the saying that "power tends to corrupt and absolute power corrupts absolutely"?[156] This phrase was coined in 1887, and although it was meant to describe absolute monarchies, it can be said about how women are treated in general—whether in society or in their homes. If someone else has power over them and over their lives, whether it is a husband or father or town elder, then unless there is some kind of check or balance, in many cases he will create conditions that are unfair and that cater to his needs instead of to her needs.

CG: I don't get it.

LL: When an individual has complete and unchecked power over another person or persons, that individual can grow insensitive to the needs and welfare of everyone. He can be cruel, steal, murder to achieve his ends because he is not subject to the rule of law. Think of the Roman Empire's Caligula who, without any government body to check his actions, visited horrible cruelty on Roman citizens.

With a kind of government that has ALL of the power—a fascist government like Nazi Germany, or what so many people in Arab countries were rebelling against in the Arab Spring…well, when a monarch has unchecked power, he is usually corrupt. You often find monarchs embezzling money and having their way with any woman they want to—without any consequences.

Who wouldn't want to be a monarch? You are basically untouched by any rule. You make your own rules. You have ALL the power. And usually when people

---

[156] The historian and moralist Lord Acton expressed this opinion in a letter to the Rt. Rev. Mandell Creighton, historian and Bishop of London, in 1887.

throughout history have had ALL of the power, what have they wanted to do — share it? No, of course not! They wanted MORE power. Look at the Roman emperors who declared themselves to be gods. Or Napoleon, who declared himself to be an emperor because king (or whatever) wasn't good enough.

Governments are not the only entities that abuse power in this way and continue to want more. Men (and some women, too) get the taste of power and also often want more. Not all men, of course, and not all women either. But many do.

CG: Yeah, but wouldn't all men — women, too — just take the power if given the chance? I mean, if they had unlimited power, they could have their wives be servants — giving them backrubs every night, and even better, giving them sex when they wanted it and on their terms. Having their wife turn into a slave whom they could slap around and order to do things…wouldn't so many men — or just people in general — do this if given the opportunity?

LL: So many people would, and that is the point. Power tends to corrupt. There are men — and women — who say they could be fair, and share and do everything right, and many of them would. But some of them would also succumb to the instinct of winner-takes-all power and do their own thing.

We need to know this about men — and ourselves — because so often women end up in abusive relationships because they did not set the ground rules from the beginning, and they did not assert their authority or power. So often women get into relationships and want to be pleasers, so they allow their partner to have more power and control, and if they are not careful, their partner will end up with an imbalanced amount. But then the woman might be stuck in the relationship and lose power because she stopped working to take care of the kids and is no longer as employable. So she becomes more dependent on her partner, and a vicious cycle starts.

Women are also at a major disadvantage in some cultures and in some countries because the laws are stacked against them. Here are four quick but telling examples:

- In Afghanistan, a woman is not allowed to decline having sex with her husband[157] unless she has a valid "excuse" or is sick. Other sections of the law allow the withholding of a woman's right to inherit her husband's wealth. Also, in the case of divorce or death, the custody of the children is decided exclusively by fathers and grandfathers.

---

[157] It's important to note that marital rape was not criminalized in North Carolina until 1984.

- In Saudi Arabia, a woman cannot get a job, go to school, or get married without the approval of her husband or father. If a woman gets a job, she must work in a women-only area, and this discourages employers from hiring women. The kingdom's religious police enforce Saudi Arabia's strict interpretation of Islam, which prohibits unrelated men and women from mingling.
- In Iran, the law says that men are guardians for women, and when a woman says a law is not fair, it is up to the clergymen to interpret the laws. The clergymen are all men and often vote against women. The penalty for not wearing a hijab (full head and body covering) is seventy-four strokes of the lash. The penalty for fornication—even if the woman is raped—is a hundred strokes of the lash.
- In the United States there is a relationship between patriarchy and rape. For example, rape is often used as a means to police the behavior of women (e.g., don't do anything by yourself, especially go out at night because you might be raped). There is a history of blaming the victim when it comes to rape and rape legal cases. Also in the United States, "Stand Your Ground"[158] laws infamously don't apply to women protecting themselves against abusers in domestic violence situations.

Every woman instinctively understands the role of power in her life and the lives of those around her. But it is not good enough if the understanding of power is buried somewhere in her brain. It needs to be brought up to the conscious mind of every woman, and it needs to be something that is well understood, dissected, and discussed. Each woman needs to understand exactly how much power she has in her primary relationships—with her spouse, boyfriend, girlfriend, or partner, and also with her in-laws, friends, parents, children, bosses, and employees. Many women do not need to do anything with this knowledge (in most cases), but they should have it.

---

158 A Stand Your Ground law states that a person may justifiably use force in self-defense when there is a reasonable belief of an unlawful threat, and the person does not have to retreat first.

When women lack power, it leads to these sad statistics:

- In Iran, forty-five women under the age of twenty were murdered in so-called "honor" killings by close relatives in Iran's majority ethnic Arab province of Khuzestan in a two-month period in 2003.[159] So-called honor defenses (partial or complete) were found in the penal codes of Peru, Bangladesh, Argentina, Ecuador, Egypt, Guatemala, Iran, Israel, Jordan, Syria, Lebanon, Turkey, the West Bank, and Venezuela (UN 2002).
- In India, there are close to fifteen thousand dowry deaths estimated per year. Dowry deaths are deaths of young women who are either murdered or driven to commit suicide by continuous harassment and torture by husbands and in-laws in an effort to extort a dowry (money or goods) from the young woman's family. Mostly, these deaths are kitchen fires designed to look like accidents.[160]
- In the United States, according to the National Center for Injury Prevention and Control, women experience about 4.8 million intimate partner-related physical assaults and rapes every year. Less than 20 percent of battered women sought medical treatment following an injury.[161]

CG: I have also heard stories about how the victims, and not the perpetrators, are often the ones punished for the crimes.

LL: Violence against women often remains unchecked and unpunished. Some countries have no laws at all. Others have flawed laws that may punish victims instead of protecting them. Even with the appropriate legislation in place, many states fail to implement the law fully.

In 2003, at least fifty-four countries had discriminatory laws against women.[162] **Seventy-nine countries have no (or unknown) legislation against domestic violence**.[163] And marital rape is recognized specifically as a crime in only fifty-one countries as far as information was available.[164]

CG: I don't understand this. If we have so much ability, and we care so deeply, then how can all of our sisters still be suffering so much, even today? Is it all because women lack power or power and privilege? And why?

---

159 *Middle East Times*, 31 October 2003.
160 *Injustices Studies*, vol. 1, November 1997.
161 Violence Against Women in the U.S.: Statistics," *National Organization for Women*, n.d., accessed November 12, 2012, http://www.now.org/issues/violence/stats.html.
162 Based on a report by the UN Special Report on Violence Against Women.
163 UNIFEM, Not a Minute More, 2003.
164 Ibid.

LL: It is a great question. In the age of the Internet, where information can be sent instantaneously and where women and men have made so, so many changes in the name of justice and morality, it is perplexing that there is still such injustice and so much pain.

Just in the past sixty years, the world has stopped Nazi Germany, and the United States has had the civil rights movement, where we went from having a culture of African Americans sitting at the back of the bus to electing our first African American president.

Women give up power, or they don't have power in the first place, and then they end up powerless or less empowered. As Roseanne Barr famously said, "The thing women have yet to learn is nobody gives you power. You just take it." That is easier said in some cultures than others.

Questions:

Do you believe that "power tends to corrupt, and absolute power corrupts absolutely"? Have you seen an example of this in your own life?

Do you think that women do not have as much power as men in your own culture? In other cultures? Why?

What are some examples of patriarchy in our culture?

Other Tragedies Being Faced By Our Sisters

LL: Sexual trafficking is also a major issue worldwide. The global market of child trafficking is over twelve billion dollars a year, and it includes one million, two hundred thousand child victims.[165] In fact, child and human trafficking is one of the fastest growing crimes in the world, and it is the second largest criminal enterprise in the world, right after drugs.

CG: That is so incredibly sad.

LL: Approximately eighty percent of human trafficking victims are women and girls, and up to half are minors.[166]

If you look at all of the conflict zones in the world, the statistics are even more startling — trafficking of women and girls was reported in eighty-five percent

---

[165] Stop Child Trafficking Now, 2012, accessed November 12, 2012, http://www.now.org/issues/violence/stats.html.
[166] U.S. State Department, http://sctnow.org/index.aspx?parentnavigationid=5812.

of the conflict zones.[167] Girls are at risk everywhere for trafficking and rape. One really sad example is that in Iraq, at least four hundred women and girls as young as eight were reported to have been raped in Baghdad during or after the war, since April 2003.[168]

While many Americans have heard of human trafficking in other parts of the world, few people know that it happens here in the United States. The FBI estimates that well over a hundred thousand children and young women are trafficked in America today. They range in age from nine to nineteen, with the average age being eleven.[169]

The Power to Make Change

LL: Laws in many countries, including the United States, do not protect women. Violence against women goes widely unreported. If you think about Lord Acton's idea that power tends to corrupt, this makes sense. Women do not report incidents of violence as much as they should because of fear of retribution, lack of economic means, emotional dependence, concern for children, and just not having access to redress. Can you imagine wanting to report a case of violence against you but knowing that if you did you might be killed or that you could endanger your children?

But that is the good thing about cultural change—when there is an injustice, usually people band together to make a change. One example of this that I love is that the women in France banded together and finally got the vote in 1945—and that was after they held out on sex nationally and forced the issue. There are all kinds of creative ways to force change to happen.

Voting is so often what gives women power in any democratic country. Unfortunately, women are way behind men in running for and getting elected to public office—we only make up eighteen percent of all elected officials in the world.[170] Perhaps if the numbers of men and women in power were more even, then the laws and conditions for women would be more in women's favor, and there would be less violence against women.

---

167 *Save the Children*, directed by Terje Rangnes, (2003: Olso, Norway: Norsk Filmfond).
168 Human Rights Watch, *World Report 2003: Human Rights and Armed Conflicts* (New York: Human Rights Watch, 2003).
169 "Teen Girls' Stories of Sex Trafficking in U.S.," *ABC News Primetime*, February 9, 2006, accessed July 2012, http://abcnews.go.com/Primetime/Story?id=1596778&page=1.
170 "Fact Sheet: Women's Political Participation, Women in Parliaments," *International Women's Democracy Center*, June 2008, accessed August, 2012,, http://www.iwdc.org/resources/fact_sheet.htm.

The good news is that there are many advocates in each country who are trying to make changes. I have come across so many examples of women in each country who are making changes—often in quite dangerous situations. They have gotten death threats, floggings, and more, but they keep on going.

CG: Could you please list them on the website? And also maybe include what we might do to help support them if they want our help?

LL: Absolutely! I will list my top heroes whose stories have inspired me on the website.

There are so many incredible organizations that help girls and women one at a time. You can probably make a significant difference in someone's life for a very small amount of money or time. For example, you can make a donation to a safe house that saves girls from forced prostitution. For only thirteen dollars a year you can help a girl stay in school in China. You can make a microloan of sixty-five dollars to give a woman in Pakistan a chance at starting her own business. You can volunteer to help with local or national or worldwide non-profit organizations. You can go online to find out about lots of opportunities. If all women who read this book got involved in just one of these causes, just think of the positive changes that we could make.

And women can help in their own country as well because *every* country has its share of issues, inequalities, and violence.

WHY SHOULD WE HELP OUR SISTERS WORLDWIDE?

Top Ten Reasons to Help Our Sisters Worldwide:

(1) <u>It is the right thing to do</u>. Martin Luther King, Jr. said, "Life's most persistent and urgent question is, 'What are you doing for others?' In the end, we will remember not the words of our enemies, but the silence of our friends."

(2) <u>Women are only as happy as our least happy vagina</u>. Our own repression as women in the West is tied in to oppression of women in the non-West. In helping others, we also help ourselves.

(3) <u>Plant a tree now, and you will provide shade for generations</u>. We are all on this earth for such a short period of time. In the scheme of things, we are born and die in a blink of an eye. We are so lucky to be given the gift of life, even if it is so short. So why don't we use the short time we

are given to make good, and send positive rays of light and energy into the world? Future generations will benefit from what we do today.

(4) <u>If you help women, you help ensure a better future</u>. When you help fellow women, they will help their boys grow into good men and their girls grow into good daughters—you will cause a ripple effect.

(5) <u>There will be less war, sadness, and killing worldwide</u>. The soul of the Universe will be happier.

(6) <u>Personal evolution</u>. The more you get out of your comfort zone, the more chance you have of evolving. Help yourself evolve and help others as well.

(7) <u>Your religion tells you to.</u> Christianity teaches "Bear one another's burdens, and so fulfill the law of Christ" (Galatians 6:2). Judaism teaches that it is a duty of Jews to "help repair the world" (Tikkun Olam). Islam teaches "Be good to your parents, to relatives, to orphans, to the needy, to neighbors near and far, to travelers in need, and to our slaves"[171]. Buddhism teaches "How wonderful it would be if all sentient beings were free of suffering and its cause! May they be free of suffering and its cause!" Hinduism teaches that one should work selflessly for the good of society.

(8) <u>But for an accident of fate, it could be your lot</u>. These women who are suffering worldwide could be our daughters, our mothers, our sisters, our cousins, or our friends. If we were in their shoes, we would want them to help us, and we would need them to help us.

(9) <u>Because you can</u>. Because if you are reading this, you likely have more resources than most women worldwide, and you likely have the ability to share with them. If not you, then who? Martin Luther King, Jr. said, "The ultimate measure of a [person] is not where he stands in moments of comfort and convenience, but where he stands at times of challenge and controversy."

(10) <u>It is quite simple</u>. As the wise Dr. Seuss said, "Sometimes the questions are complicated and the answers are simple."

---

[171] http://www.islameasy.org/K_Serving_Humanity.php

"Faith is taking the first step even when you don't see the whole staircase."

"Be the change that you wish to see in the world."

—Mahatma Gandhi

Suggested Resources:

Corrêa, Sonia, Rosalind Pethesky, and Richard Parker, *Sexuality, Health and Human Rights* (New York: Routledge, 2008).

Enloe, Cynthia, *The Curious Feminist, Searching for Women in a New Age of Empire* (Berkeley, CA: University of CA Press, 2004).

Kristof, Nicholas and Cheryla WuDunn, *Half the Sky: Turning Oppression into Opportunity Worldwide* (New York: Vintage, 2009).

Nelson, Alyse, *Vital Voices: The Power of Women Leading Change Around the World* (San Francisco, CA: Jossey-Bass, 2012).

If you care deeply about these issues and want to get involved in some way or perhaps donate money to help your sisters worldwide, please contact Vital Voices by going on to their website: http://www.vital-voices.org/.

Women Under Siege website: http://www.womenundersiegeproject.org/conflicts

My friend Janet Wagner told me about the website Women Under Siege, and I was so thrilled that she did. You can go onto these websites to find out about different parts of the world where women are under siege—you can read all about the region and what is going on. It is written in very plain language. The website is run by Women's Media Center: Amplifying Women's Voices, Changing the Conversation, and they do exactly that—in North America and around the world.

CHAPTER 21

Comfort for the Soul: Taking Care of Your Vagina *and* Yourself

LL: Women are so often the caretakers of others, so it is critical that we learn to nurture and take good care of ourselves. We can start by taking good care of our vaginas—not douching, not wearing pantiliners as often, and not dousing our vaginas with harsh chemicals. We should only share our vaginas with people who make us feel good about ourselves, and we should reevaluate our relationship with anyone who does not.

There are many other ways you should be taking care of yourself, too. Your soul, your authentic you, *needs* your care and attention. Just like on an airplane, when the flight attendant (or video) says, "In case of emergency, put on your own oxygen mask first and then your child's." This may seem counterintuitive, but if we don't take care of ourselves first, we will not have the energy to take care of others.

At the heart of all of this is that women need to believe that we SHOULD take care of ourselves. We should love ourselves, appreciate ourselves, and believe that we DESERVE to be taking good care of ourselves. If you do not feel this way, I strongly urge you to go talk to a counselor to see what is at the root of this. I also encourage you to practice cognitive behavioral therapy (Becky's triangle, see page 121) and change those negative thoughts to positive ones. Even if you need to "fake it till you make it," if you practice repeating the positive words and messages, the emotions will follow and the behaviors as well.

Here is the Vagina Revolution list of ways women should be taking care of their vaginas:

Taking Care of Your Vagina

(1) Worship your vagina! It is your life force. It does so much for you, and you need to give it some love in return.

(2) No one should ever touch your vagina unless you extend an invitation. Only allow visitors who are nice to you, good to you, and add positivity to your life.

(3) Do not douche. Your vagina is like a self-cleaning oven, and it knows how to maintain a good pH balance. When you douche or introduce your vagina to harsh chemicals, it often creates harmful conditions in your vagina.

(4) Use only products and clothes on your vagina that do not irritate. If you feel continual irritation or itching, then there is a chance you are using something that does not agree with you. What kind of pads or tampons are you using? Do you notice more irritation after wearing thongs? Have you considered that chemicals from your laundry detergent and dryer pads may be rubbing off your clothes or bed linen onto your vagina and causing irritation? Consider the idea of cutting out all potential irritants and then adding them back one by one to see if there is an obvious culprit. Also see a doctor if you have unusual irritation or itching.

> (5) Air out your vagina as much as possible. Don't sleep with underwear if you do not need to and do not overdo the pantiliners.
>
> (6) Make ALL of your days *good underwear days*. Many of us have underwear that are our favorites, and then there's the underwear we only wear when we are long overdue to do our laundry. Solution? Go out and splurge on new underwear. And throw out those old raggedy ones, and the ones with the stains from that escapee menstrual blood. You deserve it. Go to Target or Macy's or Victoria's Secret or anywhere that sells underwear—or go online to buy underwear. I, for one, am a creature of comfort and like all of my underwear to be nice and boring and comfortable, but if you like yours to be sexy or different, check out a variety of websites like FreshPair.com, VanityFairLingerie.com, and even Daily Candy has some good suggestions.

Because I am a counselor, I believe that taking care of *yourself* directly affects all of your body parts, including your vagina. Here are my suggestions for ways women should be taking care of themselves:

1. LOVE yourself and appreciate yourself. Write down a list of things you really like about yourself and keep it by your bedside. Ask your partner and friends to contribute to your list. Keep your list, along with other cards and special notes, in a special folder and keep the folder handy for occasions when you need a reminder. As Eleanor Roosevelt once said, "No one can make you feel inferior without your consent." Loving and appreciating yourself is a *choice*. Make it.

2. Appreciate others. Write a list of important people in your life and the qualities you value in them. Include your partner, children, parents, friends, colleagues, or neighbors. Remind yourself of these things often. Take the time to tell these important people why you like them and appreciate them.

3. Eat well. Research—tons of it—has shown that the way you eat absolutely affects your mood, as well as your health. Give yourself the gift of eating healthy foods that are not processed, as well as lots of fresh fruit, vegetables, whole grains, fish, nuts, and seeds.

4. It is OK to splurge. If you are going to do it, then do not feel guilty about it. It is not worth the guilt. We already have enough guilt in our lives as women.

5. <u>Choose happy, positive friends</u>. Research shows that happiness is contagious not only from your friends, but from your friend's friends as well.[172] Along the same lines, think happy and positive thoughts. There is a negative and a positive way to look at almost anything. Why not just choose positive?

6. <u>Decrease the stress in your life</u>. This will not only make you feel better, but it will also have a direct, positive impact on your health. Susan Smith Jones, author of *The Joy Factor*, points out that "two-thirds of all visits to the doctor are due to stress-related ailments, and 80 to 90 percent of all diseases are stress-related. If you control your stress, you control your immunity to disease."

This is easier said than done. One way to decrease stress is to evaluate all that you have going on in your life and put it down on paper. Rank everything in order of how important it is to you. Also indicate how much time you spend on each activity. If the two do not correlate, then work on ways to cut some things down to make more time for what is important to you.

Another way to decrease your stress is by taking a Mental Health Day (MHD) whenever you can (within reason). My college friend first taught me about MHDs when I was president of the student government association while I was an undergraduate student at Emory University. I had the habit of *all work and no play*, and she suggested that I needed to take a break. She pointed out that if I did take a break, I would be even more effective when I came back. She was right, and I have been following her advice ever since. If taking a MHD means getting a babysitter or taking a personal day from work, then DO it. Make it part of your routine, and plan one every summer — or every month — or even a few hours every week if you can squeeze it in.

7. <u>Pray</u>. If you are not religious, then *be mindful*. Send positive messages out to yourself or the universe or loved ones. This might sound corny to some women, but it does increase the positive energy in the world and in your life. Whenever I hear a fire engine or ambulance, I say a silent

---

[172] Salynn Boyles, "Happiness Is Contagious," *WebMD*, December 4, 2008, accessed October, 2012, http://www.webmd.com/balance/news/20081204/happiness-is-contagious. Research by Harvard University Medical School and the University of California at San Diego concluded that the happiness of an immediate social contact increased an individual's chances of becoming happy by 15 percent. James H. Fowler, PhD, co-author of the article reporting the study findings, said that the happiness of a second-degree contact, such as the spouse of a friend, increases the likeliness of becoming happy by 10 percent, and the happiness of a third-degree contact — or the friend of a friend of a friend — increases the likelihood of becoming happy by 6 percent.

prayer for the first responders and the people who are being affected by the emergency. I pray all day long—for my husband who is loving and so right for me, for my children, for the success and happiness of my students, for my friends who have cancer and other kinds of illness. I also send positive thoughts to anyone who is in need or who is suffering in any way.

8. <u>Think positive thoughts</u>. Buddha said, "All that we are is the result of what we have thought." Think positive thoughts and your life will follow.

9. <u>Practice Cognitive Behavioral Therapy</u> aka "Becky's triangle" (see page 121). If you don't like your response to something—whether a thought or a behavior or an emotion—then actively work on changing it. Reset your brain to appreciate more and to think more positively.

10. <u>Know when to swim upstream, but also know when to go with the flow</u>. Do you ever pick a relationship or a project, and then all you ever do is swim upstream, against all of the currents? It is just as easy to choose a relationship or a friendship where you find yourself swimming downstream—where it feels right and easy. Does your job or career make you miserable? Take career tests and figure out what would make you happier. Have to do a project? Pick the low-hanging fruit for a change to make it easy on yourself.

11. <u>If you find yourself feeling envy or jealousy (and those are normal feelings), stop to ask yourself why</u>. Jean Vanier once said that "envy comes from people's ignorance of, or lack of belief in, their own gifts." Are you not aware of your own gifts and how much they are adding to the world? Start talking to yourself more about this and concentrating on the positive. Also acknowledge the envious feelings and do not try to bury them because this only causes them to become more powerful. Acknowledge them, ask yourself why you feel this way, and work on changing these thoughts.

12. <u>Take your work seriously, but yourself lightly</u>. It is healthier if you are lighthearted and don't take everything too seriously. Your boss criticizes something at work? Take it in stride, and instead of getting angry, try to learn from it. Not having enough fun with your kids? Talk to yourself and tell yourself that they are only young once and you need to laugh more *with them* and make happy memories together. I read Gretchen Rubin's book *The Happiness Project* recently and then got one of those

one-sentence-a-day journals based on that theme, and today's date said, "It takes energy, generosity, and discipline to be lighthearted."[173] It is hard work—but well worth it.

13. <u>Be Authentic</u>. This is something that more and more women are aware of. The more a woman is true to herself, the more she embraces both her good qualities *and* her flaws, the more she learns to enjoy life and seek out the positive—and change whatever needs to be changed. The more a woman decides to focus on her *inner scorecard* rather than worry about what others may think, the happier she will be. Life is so short. Those others who you worry about will no longer be alive before you know it—nor will you! So you may as well do what *you* think you need to or should do, instead of worrying about others.

Bonnie Ware, an Australian blogger who worked for years in palliative care and is the author of the 2011 book *The Top Five Regrets of the Dying*, writes that the regret she heard most often was, "I wish I'd had the courage to live a life true to myself, not the life others expected of me."

14. <u>Celebrate Your Uniqueness</u>. It is time to be true to yourself and be yourself, no matter how kooky or strange or "out there" or wacky you are. Cast out any feelings of shame. And not only stop the shame but to embrace those differences and appreciate yourself even more for them. One of my favorite authors[174] Malcolm Gladwell has said, "Self-consciousness is the enemy of 'interestingness.'" Choose to be interesting and celebrate your uniqueness.

This is easier said than done with so many people wanting us to be something else *for them* instead of *for ourselves*. Ralph Waldo Emerson famously said, "To be yourself in a world that is constantly trying to make you something else is the greatest accomplishment." Someone who accomplished this was the late Steve Jobs of Apple. He celebrated this:

"Here's to the crazy ones. The misfits. The rebels. The troublemakers. The round pegs in the square holes. The ones who see things differently. They're not fond of rules. And they have no respect for the status quo. You can quote them, disagree with them, glorify, or vilify them. About the only thing you can't do is ignore them. Because they change things. They push the human race forward. And while some may see them as the crazy ones,

---

173 Gretchen Rubin, *Happiness Project Calendar* (New York: Workman, 2011).
174 He is my favorite author, tied with Anita Diamant who wrote *The Red Tent*.

we see genius. Because the people who are crazy enough to think they can change the world, are the ones who do."

15. <u>Seek out Personal Evolution</u>. How do you evolve? Learn about new things. Try something you want to do even if it might make you feel uncomfortable. Pursue a new hobby or career. Challenge your own thoughts about something.

16. <u>Want What You Have</u>. My close friend from high school Liz Trostler Laban always used to say, "Happiness isn't getting what you want but wanting what you have," and as I have moved many years away from high school, I have realized more and more how true that statement is.

17. <u>Everyone has a story, and everyone has something to teach you</u>. It is your job to find out what. Ask questions and then listen to the answers. Ask questions of your children, your friends, your spouse, your parents, your colleagues, and your partner. This makes people feel good, special, and validated. As the late Queen Mother said, "If you find something or somebody a bore, the fault lies in you."

18. <u>Give people the benefit of the doubt</u>. You really don't know what kind of day they have had or what is going on in their inner world. You can't possibly see other people's hardships. This also goes hand in hand with judging people less. As Mother Teresa said, "If you judge people, you have no time to love them."

But if you give someone the benefit of the doubt, and you feel that they continually take advantage of you, then reevaluate your friendship or relationship with them.

19. <u>Your life will never be perfect</u>. You will never be perfect. So you may as well learn to be comfortable with imperfection. Even love imperfection. It will take the stress out of so much.

20. <u>Be gentle with yourself</u>. I have a sign in my school counseling office that says

Be Gentle with Yourself. You Are A Child of the Universe, No Less Than the Trees and the Stars. In the Noisy Confusion Of Life, Keep Peace in Your Soul.[175]

---

[175] Ehrmann, Max, "Desiderata," 1927.

CHAPTER 22

The Word on the Word, and the Final Word

When I first started writing *Vagina Revolution* a couple years ago, I was both surprised and frustrated that vaginas—both the word and the body part—still remained in the closet.

Women were embarrassed about both the word and the body part and many women, sadly, were disassociated from their own vaginas. As a good friend of mine admitted, "I just don't think much about that whole region" as she made circular motions from her belly to mid-way down her thighs. These attitudes led to many women reporting that they were uncomfortable talking about problems or issues with their vaginas. Many women said that they were not even comfortable talking to their own doctors about their vaginas.

I sensed a need for information that would demystify and destigmatize vaginas by educating women about different aspects of them. I also thought it was important to show pictures of real vaginas—I mean, most women didn't even know what *real* vaginas looked like, except for our own. If women know exactly what other women's toes and breasts and tummies and butts and arms and abs look like, but our vaginas remain hidden, doesn't that just add to the belief that vaginas *should be* hidden?

OK, so vaginas are sort of funny looking. They have wrinkly skin and strange hair and nooks and crevices that sometimes look strange. No two vaginas are alike. Many women only see their own vaginas and then conclude that *their* vaginas are something strange, when they are really *all* so perfectly imperfect!

Many women take one look at their vagina (if ever) and conclude that it is so uncomfortable looking that they don't want to look again—and they avoid looking at it for years.

And the vaginas that women and men *do* see—usually only if they are looking at porn because where else do you find pictures vaginas—are not at all what *real* vaginas look like. They lack the beautiful asymmetry of real vaginas. They also lack the combinations of tones and colors of real vaginas—the browns fading into pinks, fading back into browns.

Somehow the porn industry has defined what a "perfect" vagina should look like, just as the fashion industry has defined what a perfectly shaped female body should look like (but that is a story for another day). And the porn industry has trained generations of porn viewers to think of *the porn versions of vaginas* as being *ideal* when they actually have nothing to do with reality. As a result, so many men have made unflattering comments to their partners, wives, or girlfriends about their vaginas or pubic hairstyle or labia length or shape—when their main point of comparison was to porn. And what happened as a result? Immeasurable women felt embarrassment or shame over their vaginas.

As if women did not already have embarrassment or shame over that body part. Countless women grew up with negative messages about their vaginas. They were *dirty* or *unsanitary*. They couldn't even have a proper name—only a nickname—because…well, why? Because the body part was so shameful it could not even be given a name?

The power of using the word vagina

There is a lot of power in using the word *vagina*. By using the correct word for the body part, women are choosing to *name* it and to *own* that body part. Language is a very important part of this whole issue.

Since I started writing this book, I have been thrilled to see that the Vagina Revolution is beginning. The word *vagina* has been mentioned much more on television and in the movies…it was featured in articles in the *Los Angeles Times* and the *New York Times*…and people are even starting to protest *not* being able to use the word in public. For example, as mentioned earlier, on June 14, 2012 a Michigan lawmaker, Lisa Brown, was banned from the Michigan House floor for using the word *vagina* during a debate on a bill that puts new restrictions on abortion providers. In response to this ban, Eve Ensler, along with Michigan lawmakers and others, planned a protest on the steps of the Michigan state capitol.

Eve Ensler spoke about why she supported this event. "For fourteen years at V-Day, we've seen the power of saying the word *vagina*. We've seen how it's freed women from their shame and empowered them to break the silence and become leaders in their communities. By saying the word *vagina* and making it OK to say the word *vagina*, we take away the humiliation, and fear, and myths that often surround it. Censoring a woman for saying a word that is a body part that fifty-one percent of their constituents have is a repression that we have not and should not ever witness in this country."

Women are ready for this change, for this paradigm shift. According to a study conducted online in August 2009 by Harris Interactive on behalf of Kotex, among more than sixteen hundred North American women ages fourteen to thirty-five, seven in ten women believe it's time for society to change how it talks about vaginal health. Yet less than half (45 percent) feel empowered to do so.[176]

If you think about it, *breasts* really just came out of the closet in the past twenty years or so. Although breasts are more front and center and easy to see, we didn't start talking about them until public health campaigns started to encourage women to do breast self-exams to check for breast cancer. Now there is a wide range of awareness and advocacy efforts, ranging from the Susan G. Komen Walk for the Cure to Save the Tatas.

---

176 Lissa Rankin, *What's Up Down There? Questions You'd Only Ask Your Gynecologist If She Was Your Best Friend* (New York: St. Martin's Griffin, 2010).

It is time for vaginas—both the word and the body part—to fully come out of the closet, and for all women to be fully knowledgeable about and comfortable with their vaginas. This book is not the start, nor is it an end. It is one step on the way to feeling good and positive about our vaginas and ourselves. We have come a long way already, thanks to extraordinary women like Eve Ensler, classic books like *Our Bodies, Ourselves,* sex researchers like Betty Dodson, and so, so many others. But there is still much more to be done. It is time for a full-blown Vagina Revolution! It is time for both the word *vagina* and the body part to be talked about loudly and proudly. Please join me at www.vaginarevolution.com to fuel the revolution, and also to find out how you can help our sisters worldwide.

Suggested Resources:

Kaufman, Gershen, *The Psychology of Shame: The Theory and Treatment of Shame-Based Syndromes* (New York: Springer, 2004).

Meston, Cindy M. and David M. Buss, *Why Women Have Sex: Understanding Sexual Motivations from Adventure to Revenge (and Everything in Between)* (New York: Times Books, 2009).

Appendices

I Personal Charting

II Which Contraceptive is Right for You?

III Sexually Transmitted Infections

IV 34 Menopause Symptoms

V Violence Against Women

Appendix 1

Personal Charting

	1	2	3	4	5	6	7	8	9	10	11	12	13	14	15	16	17	18
Period																		
Happy																		
Sad																		
Mood																		
Mood																		
Sexual																		
Pimply																		
Hungry																		
Thirsty																		
Food Craving																		
Cervical Fluid																		
Likeable																		
Energetic																		
Feeling loved																		
Gaseous																		
Poop																		
Vaginal smell																		
Body odor																		

(Continued)

	19	20	21	22	23	24	25	26	27	28	29	30	31
Period													
Happy													
Sad													
Mood													
Mood													
Sexual													
Pimply													
Hungry													
Thirsty													
Food Craving													
Cervical Fluid													
Likeable													
Energetic													
Feeling loved													
Gaseous													
Poop													
Vaginal smell													
Body odor													

Appendix 2

Which Contraceptive Is Right for You? (from the Association of Reproductive Health Professionals)[177]

Birth control methods (contraceptives) are used to prevent pregnancy. Some of them can be found at your pharmacy and some require a visit to a health care provider such as a nurse midwife, nurse practitioner, physician, or physician assistant. Contraceptives listed below with an asterisk (*) use hormones to prevent pregnancy. The contraceptive methods are in order of effectiveness with the most effective ones listed first.

Emergency contraception can prevent pregnancy after any instance of unprotected sexual intercourse. Most women can safely use emergency contraception pills, even if they cannot use birth control pills regularly. Visit www.not-2-late.com to find out where to obtain it.

Method	How to Use	Additional Information
Most Effective (typically prevents pregnancy >99% of the time)		
Abstinence/ Outercourse	Do not have vaginal intercourse	
Female sterilization: nonsurgical (Essure®) or surgical (Laparoscopy, mini-laparotomy, laparotomy)	Procedure done by health care provider	Lasts a lifetime Permanent method that cannot be reversed

---

[177] From the Association of Reproductive Health Professionals

http://www.arhp.org/Publications-and-Resources/Patient-Resources/Fact-Sheets/Which-Contraceptive

Male sterilization (vasectomy)	Procedure done by health care provider	Lasts a lifetime
		Post-procedure follow up to check sperm count is very important
		Permanent method that cannot be reversed
Intrauterine device (IUD; ParaGard®)	Inserted into uterus by health care provider	Can be used up to ten years
		Fertility will return very soon after it is removed
*Intrauterine system (IUS; Mirena®)	Inserted into uterus by health care provider	Often makes periods lighter or less painful
		Offers protection against some cancers
		Can be used for up to five years
		Fertility will return very soon after it is removed
*Implant (Nexplanon®)	Inserted by health care provider into arm	Often makes periods lighter or less painful
		Offers protection against uterine cancer
		Can be used for up to three years
		Fertility will return very soon after it is removed

Appendix 2

Very Effective (typically prevents pregnancy 91% - 99% of the time)		
*Injectables (Depo-Provera®)	Get intramuscular or subcutaneous injection monthly every twelve weeks	Makes periods lighter/less painful
		Lessens cramps
		Provides protection against some cancers & pelvic inflammatory disease
		Shot lasts twelve weeks
		Fertility may be delayed up to one year after last injection
*Pills	Swallow pill every day at approximately the same time	Makes periods lighter/less painful
		Offers protection against some cancers & breast disease
		Need to take pill every day
		Fertility will return very soon after last pill is taken
*Patch (OrthoEvra®)	Apply one patch to skin each week for three weeks in a row; then remove patch for one week	Makes periods lighter/less painful
		May protect against some cancers & breast disease
		Each patch lasts one week
		Fertility will return very soon after patch is removed

Moderately Effective (typically prevents pregnancy 81% - 90% of the time)		
Male condom (known as "rubbers")	Apply to penis immediately before sex	Provides protection against almost all sexually transmitted infections
Diaphragm	Insert into vagina with spermicide before sex	Keep diaphragm in vagina for at least six hours after sex
		Do not keep diaphragm in vagina for more than twenty-four hours
		Does not protect against HIV, but does offer some protection against sexually transmitted infections
Sponge (for women who have had a full term pregnancy)	Insert into vagina before sex	Lasts up to twenty-four hours
		Keep sponge in vagina for at least six hours after sex
		Do not keep sponge in vagina for more than twenty-four to thirty hours

Appendix 2

Effective (typically prevents pregnancy up to 80% of the time)		
Female condom	Insert into vagina up to 8 hours before sex	Provides protection against almost all sexually transmitted infections
Fertility awareness (known as "natural family planning")	Monitor cycle to determine when fertility likely/ unlikely	
Cervical cap (FemCap®)	Insert into vagina immediately before sex	
Withdrawal	Man removes penis from vagina and area near vagina before ejaculation	
Spermicide	Insert into vagina no more the one hour before sex	

Appendix 3

Sexually Transmitted Infections (from WomensHealth.gov[178])

Q: What is a sexually transmitted infection (STI)?

A: It is an infection passed from person to person through intimate sexual contact. STIs are also called sexually transmitted diseases, or STIs.

Q: How many people have STIs and who is infected?

A: In the United States about 19 million new infections are thought to occur each year. These infections affect men and women of all backgrounds and economic levels. But almost half of new infections are among young people ages 15 to 24. Women are also severely affected by STIs. They have more frequent and more serious health problems from STIs than men. African-American women have especially high rates of infection.

Q: How do you get an STI?

A: You can get an STI by having intimate sexual contact with someone who already has the infection. You can't tell if a person is infected because many STIs have no symptoms. But STIs can still be passed from person to person even if there are no symptoms. STIs are spread during vaginal, anal, or oral sex or during genital touching. So it's possible to get some STIs without having intercourse. Not all STIs are spread the same way.

---

178 http://womenshealth.gov/publications/our-publications/fact-sheet/sexually-transmitted-infections.cfm#d; U.S. Department of Health and Human Services, Office on Women's Health For more information please call 1-800-994-9662 TDD: 1-888-220-5446

Q: Can STIs cause health problems?

A: Yes. Each STI causes different health problems. But overall, untreated STIs can cause cancer, pelvic inflammatory disease, infertility, pregnancy problems, widespread infection to other parts of the body, organ damage, and even death.

Having an STI also can put you at greater risk of getting HIV. For one, not stopping risky sexual behavior can lead to infection with other STIs, including HIV. Also, infection with some STIs makes it easier for you to get HIV if you are exposed.

Q: What are the symptoms of STIs?

A: Many STIs have only mild or no symptoms at all. When symptoms do develop, they often are mistaken for something else, such as urinary tract infection or yeast infection. This is why screening for STIs is so important. The STIs listed here are among the most common or harmful to women.

Symptoms of sexually transmitted infections	
STI	**Symptoms**
Bacterial vaginosis (BV)	Most women have no symptoms. Women with symptoms may have: • Vaginal itching • Pain when urinating • Discharge with a fishy odor
Chlamydia	Most women have no symptoms. Women with symptoms may have: • Abnormal vaginal discharge • Burning when urinating • Bleeding between periods Infections that are not treated, even if there are no symptoms, can lead to: • Lower abdominal pain • Low back pain • Nausea • Fever • Pain during sex

Genital herpes	Some people may have no symptoms. During an "outbreak," the symptoms are clear: - Small red bumps, blisters, or open sores where the virus entered the body, such as on the penis, vagina, or mouth - Vaginal discharge - Fever - Headache - Muscle aches - Pain when urinating - Itching, burning, or swollen glands in genital area - Pain in legs, buttocks, or genital area Symptoms may go away and then come back. Sores heal after 2 to 4 weeks.
Gonorrhea	Symptoms are often mild, but most women have no symptoms. If symptoms are present, they most often appear within 10 days of becoming infected. Symptoms are: - Pain or burning when urinating - Yellowish and sometimes bloody vaginal discharge - Bleeding between periods - Pain during sex - Heavy bleeding during periods Infection that occurs in the throat, eye, or anus also might have symptoms in these parts of the body.
Hepatitis B	Some women have no symptoms. Women with symptoms may have: - Low-grade fever - Headache and muscle aches - Tiredness - Loss of appetite - Upset stomach or vomiting - Diarrhea - Dark-colored urine and pale bowel movements - Stomach pain - Skin and whites of eyes turning yellow

HIV/AIDS	Some women may have no symptoms for 10 years or more. About half of people with HIV get flu-like symptoms about 3 to 6 weeks after becoming infected. Symptoms people can have for months or even years before the onset of AIDS include: - Fevers and night sweats - Feeling very tired - Quick weight loss - Headache - Enlarged lymph nodes - Diarrhea, vomiting, and upset stomach - Mouth, genital, or anal sores - Dry cough - Rash or flaky skin - Short-term memory loss Women also might have these signs of HIV: - Vaginal yeast infections and other vaginal infections, including STIs - Pelvic inflammatory disease (PID) that does not get better with treatment - Menstrual cycle changes
Human papillomavirus (HPV)	Some women have no symptoms. Women with symptoms may have: - Visible warts in the genital area, including the thighs. Warts can be raised or flat, alone or in groups, small or large, and sometimes they are cauliflower-shaped. - Growths on the cervix and vagina that are often invisible.
Pubic lice (sometimes called "crabs")	Symptoms include: - Itching in the genital area - Finding lice or lice eggs

Syphilis	Syphilis progresses in stages. Symptoms of the primary stage are: • A single, painless sore appearing 10 to 90 days after infection. It can appear in the genital area, mouth, or other parts of the body. The sore goes away on its own. If the infection is not treated, it moves to the secondary stage. This stage starts 3 to 6 weeks after the sore appears. Symptoms of the secondary stage are: • Skin rash with rough, red or reddish-brown spots on the hands and feet that usually does not itch and clears on its own • Fever • Sore throat and swollen glands • Patchy hair loss • Headaches and muscle aches • Weight loss • Tiredness In the latent stage, symptoms go away, but can come back. Without treatment, the infection may or may not move to the late stage. In the late stage, symptoms are related to damage to internal organs, such as the brain, nerves, eyes, heart, blood vessels, liver, bones, and joints. Some people may die.
Trichomoniasis (sometimes called "trich")	Many women do not have symptoms. Symptoms usually appear 5 to 28 days after exposure and can include: • Yellow, green, or gray vaginal discharge (often foamy) with a strong odor • Discomfort during sex and when urinating • Itching or discomfort in the genital area • Lower abdominal

Appendix 4

34 Menopause Symptoms[179]

COMMON SYMPTOMS
1. Hot Flashes

2. Night Sweats

3. Irregular Periods

4. Loss of Libido

5. Vaginal Dryness

6. Mood Swings

CHANGES
7. Fatigue

8. Hair Loss

9. Sleep Disorders

10. Difficulty Concentrating

11. Memory Lapses

12. Dizziness

13. Weight Gain

14. Incontinence

15. Bloating

16. Allergies

---

[179] From http://www.34-menopause-symptoms.com/.

17. Brittle Nails

18. Changes in Odor

19. Irregular Heartbeat

20. Depression

21. Anxiety

22. Irritability

23. Panic Disorder

PAINS
25. Breast Pain

26. Headaches

27. Joint Pain

28. Electric Shocks

29. Digestive Problems

30. Gum Problems

31. Muscle Tension

32. Itchy Skin

33. Tingling Extremities

OTHERS
34. Osteoperosis

Appendix 5

Violence Against Women: A Fact Sheet from Amnesty International[180]

Around the world at least one woman in every three has been beaten, coerced into sex, or otherwise abused in her lifetime. Every year, violence in the home and the community devastates the lives of millions of women. Gender-based violence kills and disables as many women between the ages of 15 and 44 as cancer, and its toll on women's health surpasses that of traffic accidents and malaria combined.[181]† Violence against women is rooted in a global culture of discrimination which denies women equal rights with men and which legitimizes the appropriation of women's bodies for individual gratification or political ends.

Background

Violence against women feeds off discrimination and serves to reinforce it. When women are abused in custody, when they are raped by armed forces as "spoils of war," or when they are terrorized by violence in the home, unequal power relations between men and women are both manifested and enforced.

Violence against women is compounded by discrimination on the grounds of race, ethnicity, sexual identity, social status, class, and age. Such multiple forms

---

[180] Fact sheet accessed January 2013, http://www.amnestyusa.org/our-work/issues/women-s-rights/violence-against-women/violence-against-women-information.

[181] † UNFPA *State of World Population 2005: The Promise of Equality*. (2005), 65. UNFPA drew this figure from pp. 15 and 110 of the UN Millennium Project's *Taking Action: Achieving Gender Equality and Empowering Women*. Task Force on Education and Gender Equality. London and Sterling, Virginia: Earthscan. (2005a).

of discrimination further restrict women's choices, increase their vulnerability to violence and make it even harder for women to obtain justice.

There is an unbroken spectrum of violence that women face at the hands of people who exert control over them. States have the obligation to prevent, protect against, and punish violence against women whether perpetrated by private or public actors. States have a responsibility to uphold standards of due diligence and take steps to fulfill their responsibility to protect individuals from human rights abuses.

International Women's Human Rights Foundations

The Universal Declaration of Human Rights states that "everyone is entitled to all the rights and freedoms set forth in this Declaration, without distinction of any kind, such as race, color, sex, language, religion, political or other opinion, national or social origin, property, birth or other status" (Article 2).

The Declaration on the Elimination of Violence Against Women states that "violence against women means any act of gender-based violence that results in, or is likely to result in, physical, sexual or psychological harm or suffering to women, including threats of such acts, coercion or arbitrary deprivation of liberty, whether occurring in public or in private life" (Article 1). It further asserts that states have an obligation to "exercise due diligence to prevent, investigate and, in accordance with national legislation, punish acts of violence against women, whether those acts are perpetrated by the State or by private persons" (Article 4-c).

The Convention on the Elimination of all forms of Discrimination Against Women (CEDAW), defines discrimination against women as any "distinction, exclusion or restriction made on the basis of sex which has the effect or purpose of impairing or nullifying the recognition, enjoyment or exercise by women, irrespective of their marital status, on the basis of equality between men and women, of human rights or fundamental freedoms in the political, economic, social, cultural, civil or any other field" (Article 1).

Violence Against Women: A Human Rights Violation

Violence against women is rampant in all corners of the world. Such violence is a human rights violation that manifests itself in a number of ways, including:

▶Violence against women in custody

The imbalance of power between inmates and guards is a result of prisoners' total dependency on correctional officers and guards' ability to withhold privileges and is manifest in direct physical force and indirect abuses. Because incarcerated women are largely invisible to the public eye, little is done when the punishment of imprisonment is compounded with that of rape, sexual assault, groping during body searches, and shackling during childbirth. Women are often coerced into providing sex for "favors" such as extra food or personal hygiene products, or to avoid punishment. Furthermore, there is little medical or psychological care available to inmates. Though crimes in prison, such as rape, are prevalent, few perpetrators of violence against female inmates are ever held accountable. In 1997, for example, only ten prison employees in the entire federal system were disciplined for sexual misconduct.

▶Acid Burning and Dowry Deaths

Women's subjugation to men is pervasive in the political, civil, social, cultural, and economic spheres of many countries. In such societies, a woman who turns down a suitor or does not get along with her in-laws far too frequently becomes the victim of a violent July 20, 2005 form of revenge: acid burning. Acid is thrown in her face or on her body and can blind her in addition to [giving her] often fatal third-degree burns. Governments do little to prevent the sale of acid to the public or to punish those who use it to kill and maim. Similarly, the ongoing reality of dowry-related violence is an example of what can happen when women are treated as property. Brides unable to pay the high "price" to marry are punished by violence and often death at the hands of their in-laws or their own husbands.

▶"Honor" Killings

In some societies, women are viewed as representative of the honor of the family. When women are suspected of extramarital sexual relations, even in the case of rape, they can be subjected to the cruelest forms of indignity and violence, often by their own fathers or brothers. Women who are raped and are unable to provide explicit evidence, are sometimes accused of *zina*, or the crime of unlawful sexual relations, the punishment for which is often death by public stoning. Such laws serve to inhibit women from pursuing cases against those who raped them. Assuming an accused woman's guilt, male family members believe that they have no other means of undoing a perceived infringement of "honor" than to kill the woman.

▶Domestic violence

Violence against women is a global pandemic. Without exception, a woman's greatest risk of violence is from someone she knows. Domestic violence is a violation of a woman's right to physical integrity, to liberty, and all too often, to her right to life itself. When states fail to take the basic steps needed to protect women from domestic violence or allow these crimes to be committed with impunity, states are failing in their obligation to protect women from torture. One in four women experiences domestic violence at the hands of an intimate partner or family member in her lifetime.

▶Female Genital Mutilation (FGM)

Female genital mutilation is the removal of part or all of the external female genitalia. In its most severe form, a woman or girl has all of her genitalia removed and then stitched together, leaving a small opening for intercourse and menstruation. It is practiced in 28 African countries on the pretext of cultural tradition or hygiene. An estimated 135 million girls have undergone FGM with dire consequences ranging from infection (including HIV) to sterility. In addition, FGM has devastating psychological effects. Though all the governments of the countries in which FGM is practiced have legislation making it illegal, the complete lack of enforcement and prosecution of the perpetrators means FGM continues to thrive.

▶Human Rights Violations Based on Actual or Perceived Sexual Identity

Sexuality is regulated in a gender specific way and maintained through strict constraints imposed by cultural norms and sometimes through particular legal measures supporting those norms. The community, which can include religious institutions, the media, family and cultural networks, regulates women's sexuality and punishes women who do not comply. Such women include lesbians, women who appear "too masculine," women who try to freely exercise their rights, and women who challenge male dominance. Lesbian women, or women who are perceived to be lesbian, experience abuses by state authorities in prisons, police, as well as private actors in their family and community. Numerous cases document young lesbians being beaten, raped, forcibly impregnated or married, and otherwise attacked by family members to punish them or "correct" their sexual identity. Lesbians in the United States face well-founded fears of persecution by police because of their sexual identity and violence against lesbians occurs with impunity on a regular basis.

▶Gender Related Asylum

The UN High Commission on Refugees advocates "women fearing persecution or severe discrimination on the basis of their gender should be considered a member of a social group for the purposes of determining refugee status." (*Guidelines on the Protection of Refugee Women*) Such persecution may include harms unique to their gender such as, but not limited to, female genital mutilation, forcible abortion, domestic violence that the state refuses to act on and honor killings. However, since U.S. asylum adjudicators apply a restrictive interpretation of the international definition of a refugee entitled to protection, women seeking asylum in the United States rarely gain refugee status based on claims of gender-related violence. In particular, lesbian women seeking asylum from sexuality-based persecution in their countries of origin often, and legitimately, fear disclosing their sexuality to authorities.

The Problem of Impunity

Perpetrators of violence against women are rarely held accountable for their acts. Women who are victims of gender-related violence often have little recourse because many state agencies are themselves guilty of gender bias and discriminatory practices. Many women opt not to report cases of violence to authorities because they fear being ostracized and shamed by communities that are too often quick to blame victims of violence for the abuses they have suffered. When women do challenge their abusers, it can often only be accomplished by long and humiliating court battles with little sympathy from authorities or the media. Violence against women is so deeply embedded in society that it often fails to garner public censure and outrage.

Violence against women is a violation of human rights that cannot be justified by any political, religious, or cultural claim. A global culture of discrimination against women allows violence to occur daily and with impunity. Amnesty International calls on you to help us eradicate violence against women and help women to achieve lives of equality and dignity.

For more information on women's human rights, visit http://www.amnesty-usa.org/women or contact us at AIUSA, 5 Penn Plaza - 16th floor, New York, NY 10001 or call (212) 807-8400.

About the authors

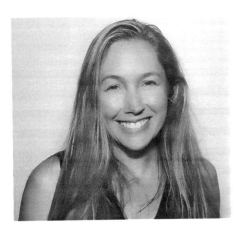

Laura Hankin Lewin is originally from New York and now resides in Charlotte, North Carolina, with her husband, Marc, and their three children aged twelve, ten, and nine. Lewin graduated from Emory University with a bachelor's degree in psychology, Duke University with a master's in public policy, and the University of North Carolina at Charlotte with a master's in counseling.

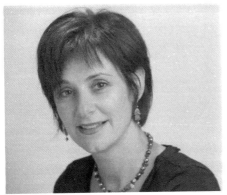

Barbara Gordon Green was born in Missouri, grew up in New York, and has lived in Charlotte, North Carolina, since 1979. She received her bachelor of arts from the University of North Carolina at Chapel Hill and her master's degree in physical therapy from Duke University. She has studied and worked extensively in the area of women's health physical therapy and sexuality for the past fifteen years. She treats both men and women with pelvic floor dysfunctions at her practice in Charlotte, North Carolina. She has two sons, aged twenty-three and eighteen.